Think of Something Quiet

A Guide for Achieving Serenity in Early Childhood Classrooms

Clare Cherry

Director, Congregation Emanu El Experimental Nursery School and Kindergarten
San Bernardino, California

Photographs by Sam Cherry

David S. Lake Publishers
Belmont, California

To my mother, Fannie Weisser,
who lived long enough to see
her noisy daughter finally
"think of something quiet."

Editorial director: Roberta Suid

Editor: Buff Bradley

Production editors: Patricia Clappison and Zanae Jelletich

Design manager: Eleanor Mennick

Designer: Hal Lockwood

Cover designer: Hal Lockwood

ISBN–0–8224–6949–9

Library of Congress Catalog Card Number: 80–82981

Printed in the United States of America

1.9   8

Think of Something Quiet

Contents

Preface   vi

Chapter One: Think of Something Quiet   1
Stress in Children   2
Dealing with Stress   3
Teaching and Learning about Stress   4
Using This Book   5
Fundamentals of a Low-Stress Program   6
Types of Movement Exercises   8
A Closer Look at the Child   10
Body Rhythms   10
Brain Hemisphere Integration   11
Tense or Hyperactive Behavior   12
Integrative Exercise   14
Rest and Relaxation for Adults   16

Chapter Two: Communicating with Children   18
Good Communication Checklist   20
Listening   22
Touching   23
Body Language   29

Chapter Three: Creating Wholesome Environments   34
Wholesome Environments   36
Color, Light, Sound and Climate   36
Bulletin Boards and Walls   37
Equipment and Furnishings   38
Room Arrangements   38
Easily Distracted Children   40
The Dual-Purpose Room   40
Quiet Places   41

Chapter Four: Responding to Stress   48
Signs of Fatigue   50
Offsetting a Fatiguing Activity   52
Loose Arrangements   53
Anticipation for Quiet   53
To Stand or to Sit   54
Muscular Exercise for Relaxation   54
Exercise After Sedentary Periods   55
Relaxation of Tension through Humor   56
Emergency!   58
Comfort for Life Crises   59
Abused and Deprived Children   63
Books   63
The Weather   64
Windy Days   65
Foggy Days   67
Stormy Days   67

Chapter Five: Getting the Most from Rest Times   70
Resting Is Not Just a "Break"   72
Short Resting Times   72
Story-Telling and Other Activities   74
Music and Songs   80
Meaningful Use of Recorded Music   80
Improvising Songs   81
Outdoor Resting Experiences   83
Creating a Restful Naptime   85
The After-Lunch Walk   86
Establishing a Routine   87
Helping Children Relax   87
Wake-Up Time   89

Chapter Six: Developing Inner Awareness   90
Heart Breathe—Techniques for Inner Awareness   92
The Value of Breathing Exercises   92

Chapter Seven: Learning to Relax Muscles   98
    Relaxation as the Opposite of Tension   100
    Isometrics and Yoga   100
    Individual Body Part Training for Relaxation   100
    Total Body Relaxation through Tension and Release   104
    Relaxation/Tension   107

Chapter Eight: Expressing Feelings to Reduce Stress 120
    An Outlet for Feelings   122
    Games About Feelings   124

    Bibliography   135

    Index   141

Preface

The conscious and unconscious anxieties which grip our daily lives are both the source and product of an increasingly complex and tension-filled society. Seeking respite from the confusion of our minds and tensions of our bodies, we turn to meditation, jogging, dancing, Yoga, hot tubs, cults, massage, biofeedback, hypnotism, and myriads of other endeavors—some commonplace and some esoteric. In our sometimes frantic search for tranquility, we often forget that children, even very young ones, are affected by the same forces which affect us, as they react to the rapid beat of society at large and to the anxious states of the adults in their personal lives.

Think of Something Quiet has been written to aid both children and adults develop skills in resting and relaxing that will help them maintain an undertone of serenity in their lives, both in and out of the classroom. The exercises and games in the book are geared to helping children learn that they can be in control of their own bodies and feelings rather than having to let their bodies and feelings control them. To this end, the book explores some of the means by which adults can enhance their sensitivity to the inner world of children and help children learn to reduce their own stress by looking inward into themselves. *Think of Something Quiet* has been developed over a thirty-year period. Hundreds of children between the ages of two and eight have shown that the games and activities are successful stress reducers. I hope they will be helpful to you.

We learn from everyone and everything. My varied experiences have brought me into contact with a great many creative and inventive persons, many of them my colleagues in teaching young children. For their ideas, inspiration, and influence I want to express my deepest appreciation. Thanks especially to my present staff who untiringly tested and helped me test the many activities in this book. Thank you Karen Ackerman, Alex Brazelton,

Margie Brown, Chuck Freidel, Kristy Garrett, Eileen Gutierrez, Susan Mercier, Linda Meyer, Karen Michaud, Cathy Rehaume, Janet Elliott-Rosengren, Saundra Shaw, Alyce Smothers, Pamela Steele, Sunny Wallick, Gary Zeidler, and Jean Zeldin. I want you to know how much help you were to me as I observed your interaction with the children and your keen sensitivities to the innuendoes of their personal actions. Your own contributions toward serenity in our interpersonal relationships have been my greatest inspiration. Thanks to you, Lois Ledbetter, Barbara Harkness, and Janet Peters, for your encouragement. Thank you Dr. Nikolai Khokhlov for your continuing dialogues with me and your faith in the scientific validity of my goals. Thanks to my two granddaughters, Deborah and Rebecca Tull, and my young friend, Sara Rosengren, for being the first to listen to many of my new stories and songs and for giving me your frank responses. And thanks to the children in the classrooms at Congregation Emanu El Nursery School and Primary Learning Center for playing the games with me, often when I interrupted your other activities. A very special remembrance to Dr. Martha Frank. And with my deepest feelings, thanks to you, Sam, my supportive husband, partner and photographer, for your insight and sharing of ideas which made the writing of this book such an enjoyable task.

Clare Cherry

San Bernardino, California

Chapter One
Think of Something Quiet

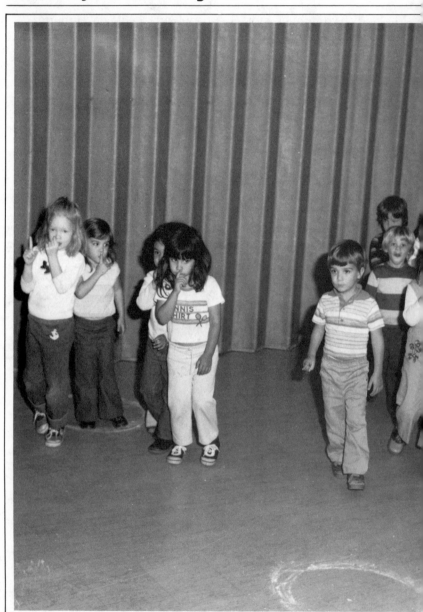

As I entered the classroom of four- and five-year olds, I was engulfed in an atmosphere of shrill, intense noise and seemingly boundless energy. I walked over to one group and said, "Look at me, everyone. I have something to tell you." As they all paused, I quickly said, in a voice barely above a whisper, "Think of something quiet. Don't tell me about it. Just think about it. I'll look at your faces and know if you're thinking of something quiet."

As each child began to grow quiet, I gave encouragement: "I can see by your faces that you are really thinking of something very quiet."

In a few moments, the classroom was silent. Slowly, deliberately, I looked directly into each pair of eyes. When I sensed a complete affinity with the group, I said, "You really know how to think of something very quiet. Now I want you to pretend you are something very quiet, to move very carefully and slowly, and to sit down on the floor near me."

We all sat quietly for a few brief moments. Then I said to the children: "Tell me with one word what the quiet thing is that you are thinking about."

In whispers, they replied, one at a time: "kitten," "pillow," "pajamas," "my cat." I repeated each of their answers, showing approval, nodding, and smiling. Then, being very careful to move quietly, I stood up and said, "You may all go back to what you were doing before I came in. Soon I'll tell you when it's time to put everything away."

The children seemed to float back to their activity areas, and within a few moments they were all busily involved in play. The atmosphere in the room was light, gentle, and relaxed, with a bit of laughter here and there.

During the next few days I paid particular attention to the interaction between the adults and the children throughout the school. The adults included experienced professionals, student teachers, parents, and a variety of volunteers. I concluded that one of their most difficult tasks was to maintain a calm, relaxed atmosphere amidst the vitality of preschool play.

Stress in Children

In planning for early childhood programs, it is important to take into account the increase in individual and group stress and anxiety which characterize our society. This stress and anxiety can result in mental and physical illnesses, mistrust and despair, and the disintegration of the family unit.

The instability of family life is probably the most serious problem young children face today. One million children a year see their parents divorced. Some of these children will live with their fathers, most will live with their mothers, and many will divide their time between two separate households. Some have the added stress of adjusting to the remarriage of one or both parents. When a parent remarries, some children acquire stepsiblings, yet another source of stress and anxiety.

The instability of the family is only one of the many factors that create stress in children. Economic pressure bears down on one- and two-parent families alike, affecting the mood and tension level in homes and schools, causing an ever-present subliminal stress. For various economic, personal, social, and political reasons, more mothers of young children are now employed outside of the home; if this situation of itself does not increase children's tensions, the attendant guilt feelings—to which many working mothers confess—certainly do breed stress in family relationships.

Large numbers of school-aged children no longer have the security of the neighborhood school to see them through their crucial first years of public education. Busing has not only removed some children from the familiarity of their neighborhoods, but has also forced children to face the added stress of long bus or car rides to schools across town.

The news media have not served children well either. The rapid-fire presentation of news events—which brings instant tragedy and disaster into living rooms—has given children distorted perceptions of human values and social mores. Advertisements and commercials create a continuous unrest by emphasizing obsolescence, dissatisfaction, and the need to acquire ever more material possessions.

Amidst these changes and pressures, parents are concerned about the growing prevalence of drug addiction and alcoholism. They also worry about whether their children will do well in school. Further, parents are concerned about their ability to protect their children from the realities and harshness of the changing society. As parents lose their own self-confidence and self-trust, they are likely to redouble their efforts to control their children, then overcompensate the severity of their behavior with extreme laxness. These wild swings between overdiscipline and overindulgence cause tremendous stress in children.

It is cause for alarm that in recent years the suicide rate for children has increased rapidly. According to figures compiled by the National Center for Health Statistics, the number of suicides committed by children ten to fourteen years old has increased by 32 percent since 1968. Child abuse is increasing at an annual rate of 15 to 20 percent, and infanticide is becoming more prevalent. A 1979 study by the American Humane Association states that in 1977, a total of 466,940 cases of child abuse and neglect were reported in the United States.

Jack Westman, in his book on *Child Advocacy*, cites a report by the 1978 President's Commission on Mental Health which estimates that 15 percent of all children now suffer from mental illness or an emotional disturbance of some type. Doctors with whom I have spoken report that children as young as six and seven years old have ulcers. Why must children in our supposedly enlightened and affluent society develop ulcers?

Children suffer stress from many other causes. Some stress is related to physical disabilities or developmental handicaps. Socially, children of minorities experience stress because of their racial, religious, or cultural differences from the majority group.

Dealing with Stress

Stress isn't always destructive. There are times when it can be beneficial. It can provide energy to meet deadlines, handle emergencies, meet challenges, and excel. But even though some stress is useful, indeed even helpful, the unrelieved, generalized stress that is pervasive in modern life is nothing but destructive to children. Children need to acquire skills that will enable them from time to time to pull back from the turmoil. They must learn how to turn inward. By turning inward I mean developing an inner awareness—an ability to find and enjoy the quietness and stillness of the inner self. If children never learn how to turn inward they may be affected adversely by unrelieved stress. It's not, however, simply a question of shutting off the external world. I tell children to think of something quiet. I tell them to think of something inside themselves—to turn their eyes inward. The desired effect is to change their attention, however briefly, from the hectic, external world to the more peaceful world of mind and thought and fantasy.

Teaching and Learning about Stress

Coursework for teachers of young children includes child growth and development; art, music, and dramatics; the teaching of reading, science, geography, history, home economics, and mathematics. Methodology classes cover such topics as creating lesson plans, charts, and progress reports; giving examinations, writing behavioral objectives, and evaluating materials. There might even be a course in child psychology that touches lightly on the discipline and control of out-of-control children.

But there aren't courses that tell you what to do when—in spite of training, carefully made plans, and a tightly organized program—children start wreaking havoc. What course explains what to do when children won't sit still, aren't interested in the lovely story being told, won't listen? Books about discipline are not the answer because they usually address the problem by telling teachers to change the child. I suggest that the problem be addressed by changing the environment and introducing children to experiences that will encourage their natural growth toward a more tranquil approach to life. Children coming into early childhood classrooms today have the right to find a casual and relaxed atmosphere in which they are treated as feeling, thinking persons who are just as vulnerable to societal conditions and tensions as are the adults in their lives. They have the right to learn the meaningful use of stress, the physiology of their bodies in relation to stress, techniques for relaxation, and the right to discover the joy of tranquility. They have the right to work and play and learn in an atmosphere of serenity, however busy their days.

By *serenity*, I mean a lack of group tension, a harmony of spirit between all members of the school community, and a high degree of inner awareness on the part of each individual. Children learn through movement, so I don't expect them to sit still for long periods of time. Children become good readers by becoming good users of language, so I don't expect them to be quiet and not talk. But I want them to know how to sit still and how to be quiet and to enjoy silence when it serves their own or the group's purpose. In other words, I want them to realize that they have the ability to control the movement or the lack of movement of their bodies and to control the stillness or lack of stillness of their minds. I want them to know that they can "turn over on their backs and float" for a while, then continue with renewed energy. I want them to know that they have the power to turn inward in order to maintain their own equilibrium.

Using This Book

Think of Something Quiet is not simply a book intended to get you a few moments of classroom quiet. It is a book that presents what amounts to a curriculum of stress reduction. This curriculum teaches children about quiet to help them understand what tension is; what it feels like; what causes it; and what they can do on their own, as well as at the instigation of their teachers, to relax tensions and ease the symptoms of stress.

Chapter Two offers teachers guidance for understanding children's stress. This understanding is actually the foundation of the psychological environment for which the teacher is responsible. Chapter Three explores the ingredients in a wholesome and restful physical environment.

The remaining five chapters present specific activities for achieving quiet, again not just to create a few peaceful moments in the classroom, but to teach children about quiet. Chapter Four suggests various ways children can respond to stressful situations in their lives. Chapter Five offers strategies for truly restful rest periods. Chapter Six is an introduction to meditative experiences. The activities in Chapter Seven seek to help children understand muscular tension and relaxation. Chapter Eight, Expressing Feelings to Reduce Stress, is, perhaps, the culmination of all that came before. It includes activities that help children, through awareness, learn to be in control of their feelings rather than allowing their feelings to control them. Children who learn this control will be able to experience more fulfilling lives in the school years and beyond.

First read the book casually from cover to cover; do not ponder too long on those parts about which you may have questions. Next, go back to the difficult parts, discuss them with others, perhaps even read some of the material in the Bibliography. Finally, select a few activities with which you will start your program. Tell the children you are just learning these games (stories, songs, exercises) yourself, and you would like them to help you. Let them help you evaluate which activities you will keep in your regular curriculum.

Fundamentals of a Low-Stress Program

The activities in this book and the suggestions for implementing them are based on a number of concepts which are essential to the establishment of a humane, wholesome play-learning program. These concepts are mutuality, self-awareness, respect, trust, caring relationships, and fantasy.

MUTUALITY
By mutuality I mean that what I want for myself, I must also want for you, and what I want from you, I must be willing to give. It might be called the Golden Rule of Awareness.

SELF-AWARENESS
More than two thousand years ago Socrates said that you must first know yourself in order to know others. That precept is just as valid today. Self-awareness is not something to cultivate just in children. It is for you as well.

RESPECT
If you want respect, you must give respect. Sometimes we forget that children deserve respect just as much as adults do.

TRUST
Trust is the basis for respect. By the time most children reach nursery-school age, they have already learned to mistrust most adults. When you show children that you are honest and sincere, that you trust them to have freedom of choice (in self-pacing and self-selection of activities), and that you will not renege on your promises, they will learn to trust and respect you.

CARING RELATIONSHIPS
People who respect each other will not allow differences to come between them. They will let differences surface, explore them through discussion, even heated discussion, and finally resolve them. The true test of our own maturity—and the modeling for children to grow toward their own maturity—comes in the reconciliation process. People who are able to confront differences and to resolve them, develop and expand their ability to care more deeply for one another.

FANTASY
Fantasy is a very real part of the world of children; it is one of their tools for coping with stress. Fairy tales, for example, carry the message that no matter how traumatic the experience, no matter how great the threat of danger, no matter how cruel a particular person, everything will work out for the best. Fairy tales and other fantasies satisfy archetypal needs within all of us; they particularly help children deal with a world that can seem hostile and threatening. I hope you will use fairy tales regularly in your classroom; tell and retell them, dramatizing them over and over again with the children. Fantasy can bring about renewed energy and a renewed capacity for achieving inner serenity.

MOVEMENT AND CREATIVE MOVEMENT

Many of the activities throughout this book are based on the creative movement of children: movement that reflects the natural developmental progress of normal children as they grow physically, and movement that gives expression to their feelings and thoughts as they grow emotionally and cognitively. (In this context, nonmovement is considered as much a part of an activity as is actual movement.)

To derive the fullest benefit from the various experiences presented, each movement should be done as slowly as possible, except when more speed is required to keep up with musical accompaniment. Try to think of movements as being soft, gentle, and quiet, and convey that feeling to the children. You should individualize exercises according to age, size, stature, body proportions, health, and experience, doing only those movements which are comfortable for each child involved. No child should force a movement. When planning movement experiences, keep environmental factors in mind—the mood of the group, the time of day, the weather. For example, on hot, muggy days you can do less vigorous activities than you'd do on cold days.

Planned movement sessions should begin, whenever possible, with a few moments of breathing exercises (see pages 92–96), and should finish with opportunities to relax with some nonmovement experiences.

In observing the degree of skill and maturity with which various children perform the movement exercises, watch for those who appear to be awkward, jerky, uncoordinated, or hyperactive, and for those who appear to have problems with spatial relationships, auditory or visual discrimination, or laterality and dominance. These children should be screened for possible developmental or physiological problems. Remediation programs should be undertaken to assist them toward normal development.

Types of Movement Exercises

The movement experiences throughout this book incorporate specific categories of movements. By understanding these categories, you can expand the curriculum with variations and additions of your own.

WHOLE BODY MOVEMENTS
Whole body, nonlocomotor movements are done from a sitting or standing position and do not transport the body from place to place. Typical whole body movements include bending, stretching, wiggling, shaking, swaying, rocking, twisting, bouncing, and gesturing.

LOCOMOTOR MOVEMENTS
Locomotor movements move the body from place to place and involve such basic skills as walking, running, jumping, leaping, hopping, crawling, creeping, sliding, rolling, climbing, skipping, and galloping.

FINE MOTOR MOVEMENTS
Fine motor movements incorporate the use of small muscles necessary, for instance, in doing artwork.

BILATERAL MOVEMENTS
Bilateral movements involve both sides of the body equally. For example, clapping hands is bilateral; waving is not.

UNILATERAL MOVEMENTS
Unilateral movements involve only one side of the body at a time, such as hopping on one foot, waving, or standing on one foot. Bear in mind that a two-, three-, or four-year-old may be working just as hard to control the side that is not in use as the one that is. For example, while hopping on one foot, holding one knee bent may be just as difficult as getting the other leg off the ground.

CROSS-LATERAL MOVEMENTS
Cross-lateral movements involve both sides of the body by alternating the movements of opposite body parts, as in walking and running. When one leg goes forward, the other goes back while the opposite arms go forward and back at the same time. Young children who can creep on their hands and knees or crawl flat on their stomachs cross-laterally, have achieved balance, body control, a measure of self-awareness, laterality, dominance, and

hemisphere integration. (Many young children with learning disabilities can be helped to lessen those disabilities by efforts to develop cross-laterality.)

The goal of all these kinds of movements is the balanced, natural development of the child. Retarded or imbalanced development is a source of tremendous stress in children. When children develop naturally, stress is kept to a minimum.

A Closer Look at the Child

It's important for the teacher to be sensitive to the psychological circumstances, the "inner weather," of each child, and to understand and respond to stress-related behavior.

Body Rhythms

The unique temperament and personality that each of us has is in part due to bodily rhythms that determine, among other things, the pace at which we function, our needs for sleep and nourishment, and our cycles of activity and rest and energy and fatigue.

Just as temperament and personality vary widely from individual to individual, so do body rhythms. In planning relaxation and resting activities for groups of children, you must pay attention to their individual differences. For instance, you should try to identify those children who have higher energy levels and give them some extra physical activity from time to time. And those children who seem to fatigue more easily may need frequent motivation to participate in quieting and relaxing activities.

Certain regularities in your program are important. There should be a very regular schedule for eating and napping. But there should also be enough flexibility in play and study times so that children can learn to know their own rhythms within those times. Open-ended programs can allow for children who need to nap earlier or later than others; for children who need frequent opportunities to rest in a quiet place; for children whose blood sugar function requires them to have frequent, small snacks; for children who need to use the toilet frequently; and for children who are so lethargic that they need frequent and extraordinary stimulation.

Brain Hemisphere Integration

In most people, the right hemisphere of the brain controls the left side of the body, and the left hemisphere controls the right side. Other functions of the two sides are quite different. The right hemisphere normally controls spatial and postural factors that pertain to how we learn to move and navigate through space. It is also the source of such elusive phenomena as intuition, artistic expression, recognition of faces, body image, fantasy, and imagination. The left hemisphere is primarily the source of analytic and logical thinking, verbalization, mathematical ability, and sequencing. Because of the strong emphasis placed on language and quantitative thinking in our society, especially in our traditional systems of education, we tend to neglect the functions of the right hemisphere and overemphasize the left.

In our work with young children, it is important to develop activities that emphasize the functions of both hemispheres in order to help children find balance, harmony, and control within themselves.

The activities in this book seek to develop the responsiveness of the right hemisphere through the use of imagery and imagination, fantasy, color, spatial relationships, and other sensory input. The activities also exercise the left hemisphere by using language, sequence, logic, design, and color. The brain uses the responsiveness of the right hemisphere and combines it with the organizational and ordering ability of the left hemisphere to achieve integrated functioning. When left–right hemisphere integration has been achieved, there is less stress within the individual. This results in a greater ego strength and self-awareness and in an increased ability to relax tensions and to control the body and the mind.

Tense or Hyperactive Behavior

One of the problems in expanding the opportunities for relaxation and inner awareness in early childhood classrooms is that there may be two or three children who demonstrate unusual tension, hyperactive behavior, or both. These children should not be taken for granted. Research during recent years has led to new findings about the causes of such behavior and has suggested new approaches in helping such children.

Just as people are physically and psychologically unique, they are also biochemically unique. Substances that most persons can tolerate may prove intolerable to others. Take sugar for example: In some extremely sensitive children, even the smallest amount of sugar, including honey and brown sugar, will cause an allergic reaction which may set off hyperactive behavior.

Extremely large amounts of sugar will cause almost all children to be temporarily overactive and noisy for a period of time lasting from one-half hour to two or more hours. You can see the effects of sugar at the typical birthday party when, after refreshments, parents wonder with despair why their previously well-behaved children go wild. The same children, attending a party in which the refreshments are nuts and raisins, or popcorn and apples, will continue more relaxed social behavior for the duration of the party.

Lendon Smith explains in *Improving Your Child's Behavior Chemistry*, that the sugar reaction is caused by a disturbance in the body's blood sugar level. The ingested sugar temporarily increases the flow of insulin. The increased insulin raises the blood sugar to a level which stimulates increased activity. This increased insulin so overworks the pancreas that suddenly the level of insulin is depleted, and the blood sugar drops below normal. It is at this point that the child's behavior may become bizarre as the body tries to balance too much one moment and too little the next.

Protein has somewhat the opposite effect of sugar. Protein does not burn as quickly as sugar and will raise the blood sugar just slightly; this means that the insulin is not used up so fast that the pancreas becomes depleted. Nuts and cheeses make good protein snacks to offer children in place of sweets.

In *Why Your Child Is Hyperactive*, Ben Feingold explains that some persons are allergic to certain food additives such as preservatives, flavorings, and colorings. These additives can cause symptoms of hyperactivity. If you suspect that such might be the case for a particular child, suggest to the parents that they implement an absolutely controlled diet for a few days— no artificial substances of any kind in foods. If there is an obvious improvement in the child's behavior, you might recommend that the parents contact the nearest Feingold Society where they can get information about a permanent, additive-free diet. For the name of your nearest branch, write to the National Health Federation, P.O. Box 688, Monrovia, CA 91016.

Other chemicals may be ingested with foods or absorbed from the polluted environment; these chemicals can also cause hyperactivity in children. An analysis of the percentage of chemicals in a child's body may indicate lead or cadmium poisoning, or may indicate a chemical deficiency that can lead to overactivity and other behavioral problems.

Sometimes hyperactive, disruptive, or tense behavior is due to underdeveloped or unevenly developed sensorimotor and perceptual-motor skills. *Underdevelopment* means a child is maturing more slowly than the average child, but is doing so in a normal sequence. Such children, whether smaller than average in size or not, have less than average ability to perform motor tasks. These children may sometimes appear lethargic rather than overactive. But they frequently have a great deal of inner tension and anxiety, and they need much help in developing self-awareness and ease of movement.

Unlike slow developers, children with *uneven development* may have skipped one or more stages in the normal growth sequence; they suffer from frustrations and tensions due to the resulting imbalances.

Children who are slow developers or who develop unevenly can be identified by simple screening of their motor abilities, sensory awareness, and perceptual-motor skills. Children who are awkward, clumsy, seem to be confused about direction, fall frequently, or bump into people or things ought to be checked for developmental problems. Also check those who are bright and/or athletic but have difficulty recognizing their names or handling small manipulative tools such as scissors or crayons, and otherwise demonstrate problems with eye-hand coordination. Not all of these children display hyperactivity, but many are aggressive and anxious. Some have such poor self-images that they may cry frequently and easily, or may become completely withdrawn. As children go about their play, notice if they have difficulty with such simple motor activities as walking, running, hopping, climbing, balancing, and crawling. If children have difficulty with several of these, further testing is indicated. (For further information, refer to the Bibliography.)

It has been my experience that children who are underdeveloped or unevenly developed are frequently helped to function more harmoniously and serenely by deep involvement in the kinds of activities that are emphasized throughout this book. These activities can lead to inner awareness and control of body and mind.

Integrative Exercise

One activity that I've found particularly helpful for slow and/or uneven developers is the Flip-Flop Game.

Susie was a talkative, intelligent, and attractive youngster. At four-and-one-half years of age she was bright and well liked. She knew how to print her name, but always made the two s's backwards. I tested Susie and found her to be immature in several areas of perceptual-motor development. Then I taught Susie the Flip-Flop Game. After this exercise, Susie would make her s's correctly for the next twenty minutes or so. She moved around the room more rhythmically and was graceful in her actions. She gradually slipped back into her casual clumsiness. For Susie, many other remediation techniques were used, and eventually she increased her perceptual-motor skills to normal functioning. Meanwhile, I began using the Flip-Flop Game with other children who were four-and-one-half years old or older. Their teachers noticed that this simple integrative exercise had a calming effect on the children. First- and second-grade children were better able to concentrate and to follow directions on academic assignments after their daily five-minute session playing this game; they appeared more relaxed and free of tension.

The Flip-Flop Game is based on the natural sleep position of human beings. It puts children through the same type of movement pattern which infants experience when they first begin crawling. Many years of experience with this exercise in the normal early childhood classroom has led me to include it as part of a daily program of relaxation games.

◥ The Flip-Flop Game

Ask children to lie face down, assuming the position illustrated in the photograph below. Study the photograph carefully to help children learn the correct position. Fingers should point straight ahead when the elbow is bent. The elbow and knees are bent at right angles. To help beginners get started, I say, "Pretend you're a little baby wanting to suck your thumb, but you can't get the

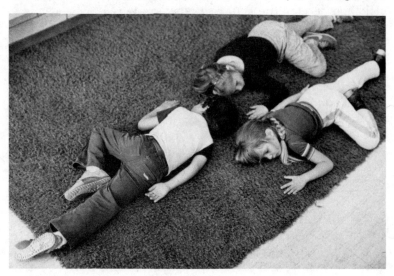

thumb next to your mouth." Some children, especially those with perceptual problems, may need a lot of help at first in doing the exercise.

It doesn't matter which direction children face. Right-handed children will usually face to the right and left-handed children will face to the left. Once children are in the correct position, the teacher says, "Flip." The children take the same position but face in the opposite direction. Then the teacher says, "Flop," and the children move back to their original positions. In making the movements, children should be reminded to keep as much of the body in contact with the floor as possible.

Rest and Relaxation for Adults

The adults in the school community must be given just as much opportunity for rest and relaxation as the children. Remember that the casual and relaxing environment you help create for children will benefit you as well. You should participate in the relaxation and awareness exercises included in this book; they'll help you develop the ability to relax tensions at will, as well as to discover the restful benefits of looking inward.

Planned breaks are important. There must be a place in which you can close off the sounds of the classrooms and play areas, and spend a short time reading, knitting, drinking a cup of coffee, writing letters, or just resting. (In business and industry such breaks have been shown to increase efficiency, diminish the number of accidents, and improve interpersonal relations between employees.)

There should be a built-in plan to allow the school's adult community to socialize without being concerned about supervising children at the same time. Teachers can get isolated and lonely in their jobs, thus adding to their stress load. Break periods ought to be scheduled so that two or more teachers can have breaks together. I like to plan the first fifteen or twenty minutes of a staff meeting for social exchange, and once in awhile even devote an entire meeting only to that purpose. Birthday celebrations, special events, and prevacation parties are good opportunities for staff members to socialize.

Finally, take care of your emotional and physical health. Learn to express your feelings so that they don't get all bottled up, creating ever-growing tension and stress. Practice relaxation exercises to help you cope with the tensions generated by work and by personal problems. Remember: No matter what the school environment, the background of your children, or your job description, the greatest single factor in helping children learn about relaxation is *you.*

Chapter Two
Communicating with Children

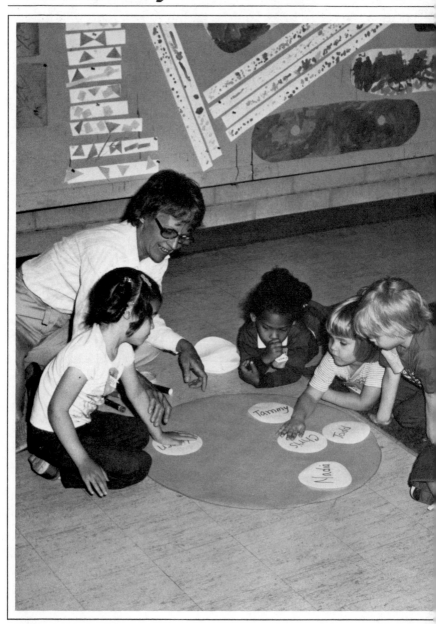

As the children entered my room one day, I greeted each one individually from where I was sitting on the floor. I invited them all to join me. I had a large, circular piece of white paper and a handful of colorful marking pens on the floor next to me. I said to each child in turn "I'm glad you're here. I'll put your name on this paper so everyone will know you're here. Where would you like me to put your name?" Each child pointed to a place on the paper.

I continued: "What color would you like me to make your name?" Then I carefully printed the child's name in bold, important-looking letters.

After everyone had arrived, I placed the name-circle on the bulletin board, low enough so that these three- and four-year-old children could touch it. From time to time, during the ensuing hours, various children went to the bulletin board to point out their names. A number of times during the day, I went to the name-circle and repeated all of the names.

This activity let the children know that I was honestly glad that they were there—not simply because I had said so but because I found an even more effective way to communicate appreciation of their presence.

Contributed by Sunny Wallick

Good Communication Checklist

There are many ways to communicate with children. When I say, "Think of something quiet," I am verbally communicating a request for something I want them to do. By the tone of my voice, by my posture (stance), and by my facial expressions and gestures, I am also communicating something about how I feel and what I am thinking. There are many indications that children intuitively receive messages even when the sender is not aware of the communication. Our concerns here, however, are those normal, everyday ways in which, by being aware of how we are communicating, we can improve communication and promote a more serene kind of human interaction.

Here are some suggestions that will help children to be relaxed and comfortable in response to the way you communicate with them (and thus, the way in which you model methods of communication):

- Take plenty of time. Don't rush children (unless an emergency exists). Don't be impatient. Relish each extended moment that you are privileged to interact with others.
- Show children that you are aware of their presence. When speaking to children look directly at their faces; don't talk over their heads or behind their backs. When talking to children, touch them whenever possible. Lean forward toward them.
- Let children know that you appreciate their presence. Hug. Pat. Smile. Nod frequent approvals. Don't hesitate to say out loud, "I'm glad you are here," or "I'm happy to see you. I really am." Be sincere. Get down to their eye level whenever possible.
- Listen. Listen. Listen. Let children finish what they are telling you. Be patient. Give encouragement. Tell them it's all right to take their time. Listen not only to the words but to the whole message. Children sometimes have difficulty getting their real meaning across to you.
- Give children instant feedback by repeating or rephrasing what they tell you. That way, if you have interpreted the

message differently from what they intended, they have an opportunity to correct you. Ask, when uncertain, "Is this what you are trying to tell me?" Communication is blocked unless there is a clear understanding by both parties involved.

- Modulate your voice. Be clear and precise; don't talk loudly, too quickly, or too roughly. Use gentle expressions as often as possible, with variations of tone. Sincerity, not volume, will make children more apt to listen and accept what you are telling them.
- Help children to talk about themselves, their families, their homes, their activities, and their feelings. Accept what they tell you without judgment. Learn to enjoy the uniqueness of each child.
- Be relevant when communicating with children. Use simple words, and talk about things within their areas of understanding and experience. They can learn new words in stories and songs, but in your day-to-day conversations with them, simplicity is the key.
- Let children know that you are aware of and appreciate their personal lives, their backgrounds, and their families.
- Develop trust by showing children that they can trust you to be honest, caring, and sincere. Always follow through on promises, if possible, but don't be afraid to apologize and say you've made a mistake and have to change a plan or a promise. Develop trust by always showing children respect and helpfulness.
- Don't make assumptions about what children are thinking or feeling. If you really don't understand, say so. Also, talk with others—teachers and parents—who can help you understand. Be sure you understand children's messages before you act.
- Give constant encouragement.
- Have realistic expectations and let the children know, honestly, what those expectations are.
- Show children your appreciation for little accomplishments, successful relationships, and even just their presence in the room.

- Always remember that your facial expressions, gestures, and postural attitudes communicate more to children than any number of words you might say.
- Touch children often. Touching is a universal means of communication and is especially effective when interacting with children.
- Avoid: using a loud voice; yelling and screaming; giving commands rather than making requests; putting others down; ignoring; being indifferent; being too busy to give time and attention, or to listen; teasing or shaming; being demanding; threatening; bribing; lying; cheating; breaking promises; being prejudiced; and being incongruous and inconsistent.

Three of the points on the good communications checklist are important enough to demand further discussion. They are listening, touching, and body language.

Listening

Listening is a two-way process. The listener also needs to be listened to. Listening isn't always easy. Our lives are permeated with artificial sounds from traffic, household appliances, radio and television sets, telephones, factories, trains, and aircraft. For self-protection, children, and many adults, learn to turn off much of what they hear. This turning off may cause perceptual difficulty in differentiating between primary and background sounds.

As the teacher, you have a responsibility to model appropriate listening behavior so that the children can learn from you. The art of listening requires a nonjudgmental approach, with attention focused completely on the person to whom you are listening. You must show a willingness to receive the information without making predetermined conclusions.

Interpretation must be in the context of what the children's perceptual and cognitive development tell you they are meaning, rather than what the actual words are. For example, "Daddy will get me pretty soon," is not a statement of fact, but a request for reassurance from the adult. When Rebecca says, "I'm up high," she means for you to comment on the fact that she is getting taller. When Julie says, "I'm empty," she is telling you that she is hungry and that she wants you to assure her that she will eat soon. A more difficult situation to decode happens when Rod comes to you and says, "But I had the truck first and Bobby is mean." Listen carefully. He may be telling you that he has just socked Bobby and that Bobby is probably on his way to you with tears streaming down his face. Your job is to determine (without cross-examination) (1) whether Bobby took the truck from Rod, or (2) whether Bobby had the truck first, Rod had taken it from him, and Bobby was just trying to get it back.

Trying to be nonjudgmental, in such a case, I would probably say, "You both look very unhappy, but I don't want to get involved in your argument. You and Bobby discuss it; listen carefully to each other, and you will be able to figure out what to do." The key is in telling them to listen to each other. Usually, if you have modeled good listening habits yourself, such an incident will end up with the two children deciding to play together happily and cooperatively.

The listening you do can be a demonstration of trust. Trust is the result of respect. You listen to Rod respectfully and non-judgmentally, you respect Rod and Bobby as individuals, and you respect their right to quarrel; at the same time you respect their ability to understand your not wanting to get involved. Your modeling helps them to respect each other.

Touching

Touching is both a primary means of communicating with children and a primary means by which children communicate with each other and with adults. Some studies have shown that children who have been touched with much care and tenderness during their infancy, and have continued to receive much careful touching during toddlerhood, learn to be gentle and trusting in both giving and receiving messages through touch. But children who have not been touched much during infancy, or who have been treated carelessly and roughly, may develop an outright fear or avoidance of touching others (or of being touched by others), or they may do so carelessly and roughly.

The mutuality of human interaction and the ability to relax in a group situation can be enhanced through increasing the comfort and ease with which people touch each other. It is important to give children exercises that increase their awareness of touching, their sensitivity to touching, and their ability to control the ways in which they touch each other. Such experiences are crucial to achieving a tension-free environment.

First you should develop the habit of touching children as frequently as possible. Look for those myriad opportunities when the touch of your hand can say more than any number of words. Next, introduce the children to simple touching games, such as the ones that follow. Often children will touch one another roughly until taught to do otherwise. Instead of saying, "Keep your hands to yourself," say to the children, "Touch softly," or "Touch gently," or "Touch so it doesn't hurt." Tell them you are going to play some games that will help them learn how people like to be touched. After such games, it's helpful to evaluate them with the children. Ask children what their feelings were, what parts they liked best, what they didn't like. Their particular answers aren't as important as the awareness such questioning creates.

◄§ Hand Squeeze

Children frequently hold hands for circle games. Children and adults frequently shake hands as a form of greeting. Yet, hand-holding and hand-touching is taken very much for granted. The following exercise can serve to increase the importance of hand-touch to everyone involved, thus enhancing interpersonal communication skills.

1. Ask everyone to form a circle (sitting or standing) and to hold hands.

2. You begin by gently squeezing the hand of the child to your right, then relaxing your grip.
3. That child then squeezes the hand of the next child to the right, then relaxes.
4. Continue around the circle until everyone has squeezed the left hand of the person to the right.
5. Repeat, but reverse the procedure, going to the left.
6. Do a few group squeezes in unison. You can say, "Hold. Squeeze. Hold. Squeeze," for whatever length of time seems appropriate.

◆§ Shake My Hand

In playing this game, children three and under can stand in a random grouping; older children can form a circle. Before starting the game, demonstrate the proper way to shake hands. You might first have everyone shake hands with you and then with each other. Remind them not to pull, push, poke, squeeze, yank, or otherwise manipulate others. Rather, they are to grip hands, squeeze gently, and then let go.

SHAKE MY HAND
(Tune: "Oh, Susannah)

Oh, I like to say hello, hello,   Holding hands going in a circle.
   It means how-do-you-do.
Oh, I like to say hello, hello,   While holding hands, everyone goes
   To you, and you, and you.   towards center of circle. Clasped hands are thrust out and touched one to another.

Chorus:

Hello in the morning, hello everyone,   Children shake hands with
We'll sing and play and work and dance,   person on right, then with
And have a lot of fun.   person on left.

Sing the song again, substituting *shalom, aloha, hola,,* and so forth, for *hello.*

Discussion:

1. Besides using words, what other ways are there for people to say hello to each other?

2. How do you feel when someone comes into a room and doesn't notice you?
3. How do you feel when someone notices you but doesn't say hello?
4. Why is it better to shake hands than to just say hello?

HOW DO YOU DO, MY PARTNER
(Tune: "Lazy Mary Will You Get Up")

Have the children select a partner and stand facing each other; they should change partners for each new verse.

How do you do, my partner, my partner, my partner?
  How do you do, my partner, my partner today?   Shake hands.
I rub your hand my partner, my partner, my partner,
  I rub your hand my partner, my partner today.   Rub each other's hands.

Other verses
I pat your cheek my partner
I rub your arm my partner
I pat your back my partner
I bump your hip my partner   Bump with hips.
I clap your hands my partner   Clap as in "Patty-Cake."
I swing your arms my partner   Hold hands, swinging arms.
I give a hug my partner
I back-to-back my partner   Bump with buttocks.
I shoulder-bump my partner   Bump with shoulders.

✺ To Touch a Star

For developing group harmony, use this gentle touching exercise that delights young children. Start the activity by having everyone sing with you, very softly, "Twinkle, Twinkle, Little Star." Then tell the children that you know how they can touch a star. Do the following activities with six to eight children in a group, holding each position for one minute.

1. Have each group of children form a loose circle with everyone facing sideways, in the same direction, so that the right arm is toward the center of the circle.

2. The children stretch their right arms toward the middle of the circle. If the hands do not touch, have everyone move inward, until hands can be held in an overlapping position, one on top of the other. This is the basic "touching star."

3. Now have everyone take one or two more slides (sideways) toward the center. Keeping their elbows stiff, and not changing the position of their hands on top of each other's, they can raise their arms toward the ceiling. This is the "high touching star." When they have achieved this position, give the following suggestion: "Let's all stand very still and quiet. Just let yourself be the beautiful, sparkling, bright-shining, touching star."

Variations on the basic To Touch a Star activity can be introduced slowly. Start by having children learn one or two variations, and when these have become familiar, add one or two more. Finally, when you have had a chance to try all of the methods, select for regular use those that the children showed the best response to, and eliminate the others. You might ask children to help by naming their favorites.

✌§ *Low Touching Star*

The "low touching star" is similar to the "high touching star" formation in the original exercise, except that the arms are extended downward toward the floor rather than upward toward the ceiling.

✌§ *Jumping Star*

For the "jumping star," have the children hold the first position of touching hands. The child whose hand is at the bottom of all of the other hands brings it around and places it on top. The child whose hand is now at the bottom repeats the action. Continue until the hands are back in their original positions.

✎ Falling Star

The "falling star" is similar to the basic "touching star" formation, except that each child stretches one leg toward the center of the circle. When all toes are touching, it is the "falling star."

✎ Double Stars

Everyone holds hands in a loose circle, facing toward the center. Children stretch their arms out in front toward the center of the circle, while still holding each other's hands. Everyone takes one slow step at a time toward the center until all of the clasped hands are touching each other. "Double stars" can be made into "high double stars" or "low double stars."

✎ Cluster Stars

For "cluster stars," children form a circle with right feet pointed toward the center. They bring their right arms over their heads and down in an arc until they can clasp their ankles. In this position they may have to move toward the center very slowly until they feel the touch of one another's heads. This is a difficult exercise, but it's one that gives much satisfaction to the children.

✎ Designing Stars

Children lie down on the floor in a circle with their heads toward the center. They stretch their arms over their heads until their fingertips are touching each other's. Ask everyone to close their eyes and think how it feels to be part of a "star design."

✎ Sleeping Stars

The "sleeping star" is similar to the "star design" formation, except that only one hand reaches to the center. The other one is used to cushion the head. Say:

Pretend that you are a bright, twinkling, faraway star. Your shine is so beautiful that people on earth keep looking and saying how good it makes them feel to look at you. Inside of your head you can try to see all of the bright lights of all of the other stars. How still and quiet they all are. So still. So quiet. So beautiful. So bright. So very, very quiet.

You can also do individual "sleeping stars" using the following introduction:

Find your own place somewhere in this room. Pretend the room is the sky. Now, make yourself into a beautiful sleeping star.

Continue as above with "Your shine is so beautiful. . . ."

WAKING, WAKING, LITTLE STAR
(Tune: "Twinkle, Twinkle, Little Star")

Waking, waking, little star,
Stretching as you shine so far,
Stretching out your shining light,
Shining in the sky so bright,
Waking, waking, little star,
Stretching as you shine so far.

Body Language

Timmy's mother enters the building, rushes to sign him in for the day and glances impatiently at her watch. "That kid," she says. "I'm going to be late again." And here comes Timmy, shuffling slowly into the room, his shoulders slightly slouched forward, his arms dangling loosely at his sides, and his head bowed down. Recognizing that he has already been defeated by the adult world before the day has hardly started, I greet him with a hug, feeling his body blend into mine. "I'm so glad you're here," I say. I squeeze his hands and add, "It always makes me feel good when you come to school." He smiles shyly at me, lifts his head, and walks to his classroom.

A few moments later, Ruth comes storming into the room ahead of her father. Her fists are clenched, her shoulders are tilted, and her chin is jutting forward. Defiance defines her entire demeanor, and it's easy to see she's out to get me or anyone else who gets in her way. By the look of frustration and discouragement on her father's face, I can recognize that they've been battling. He appears to be so embarrassed that I reassure him, "We're really planning a special surprise today. She'll be all right. Please don't worry." He smiles at me in relief, shakes his head, and turns to go, muttering, "Well, some days . . . I just don't know. . . ." But he walks just a little straighter than when he arrived. With Ruth's father on his way out, I put my arms out toward Ruth, whose body stiffens as I draw her to me. "Some days everything is all wrong," I say. "I can tell you're not having a good morning, are you?" Although her body remains tense, her shoulders slacken a little, her jutting chin falls back into place, and she glances at me quizzically. I smile, nod my head, and say, "I'm really glad you're here, Ruth. I really am." She relaxes just a little, hesitates, then suddenly skips off to her classroom.

When I tell these children "I'm glad you came today," they can tell from my facial expression and the touch of my hands, much more than by my words, that I really mean what I say. I do mean it. The children are the reason I have the job I have. Their attendance, and their attending moods, are very important to me.

Verbalization actually comprises only a small percentage of the messages human beings send to each other during any period of interaction. By heightening your awareness of the many facets of nonverbal communication that are constantly influencing actions and reactions, you can extend the potential for a tension-free environment. Learn to watch how children enter the room. Are their heads held high and their backs arched with confidence, or do they move haltingly and hunched with fear, defeat, or discouragement? Do they stand as though their world were all askew, or are they straight and at ease? Do they turn away in boredom or disinterest, or do they lean forward eagerly with alertness and anticipation? Watch for signals conveyed by postures, movements, and gestures. For example, hands brought to the mouth might mean astonishment or wanting to make an apology. Crossed arms may indicate defiance or stubbornness. Clenched fists and pouting lips can indicate anger. The clues are many. Watch for them, evaluate the accompanying situation, and respond to them. By responding appropriately, you can help alleviate the pressure of certain moods and feelings before they deteriorate into out-of-control episodes.

Nonverbal communication works two ways. Children are affected by your body language probably even more than you are affected by theirs. Be cautious about sending double messages— messages in which you say one thing with words, but by your demeanor, the look on your face, or your stance, you convey something other than what the words are saying. When you are being completely honest with children, your words and your body language will complement each other. When you're saying what you don't mean, words and body language will conflict. Children will either get the real message, no matter what you've said, or they will be very confused by the double message.

✍ Nonverbal Conversations

To promote feelings of mutality and to enhance interpersonal relationships, you can introduce some classroom activities to help children become more aware of the importance of body language. After participating in activities similar to those that follow, you can further increase their value by involving the children in discussions about what took place. Ask them questions such as:

Did you like talking without saying words out loud? Why? Why not?

What was the hardest part of getting other people to understand you?

What was the easiest thing to tell other people without using words?

Did you like the quiet in the room or do you like it better when everyone is talking? Why?

What would you do if you were in a place where no one

could understand the words you were saying? How would you be able to tell other people what you needed? What would you do if you had never learned how to talk? What are some of the ways your hands can talk for you? What are some of the ways your eyes can talk for you? What are some of the ways your body can talk for you?

✌ I'm Talking to You

Have the children group themselves into pairs. Let them play some games, puzzles, build with blocks, or do whatever activities are available in the classroom. Tell them that they can only talk with each other through body language; everyone is to be silent.

✌ Thanksgiving Children

During the time of the Pilgrims, children were not allowed either to talk or to sit at meals. One day, have the children stand around their tables while eating lunch. Everyone must remain absolutely silent. If some children normally do not bring lunches, or if lunches are not provided at school, plan a special day when everyone has a midmorning lunch or stays a half hour later to eat a sack lunch brought from home.

✌ Silent Hour

Select one hour during a normal school day when everyone, including the adults, is to be silent. Communication will only be allowed through the use of body language.

✌ Charades

Charades is the classic body-language game. Divide the children into two teams. The first team acts something out while the second team tries to interpret it. When the second team guesses the answer, it takes its turn acting out, and the first team guesses the answer.

✎§ Pantomime

Have one or more children interpret a poem, rhyme, song, play, or whatever else you choose to read for them, by acting it out. After several performances, the children will be able to pantomime familiar verses or stories without having them read aloud.

✎§ Pantomime to Records

Pantomime to records is not only a good body-language exercise but also an excellent way for children to develop listening and language skills. Select a recording of a familiar song. Have everyone "sing" to the record, but silently, mimicking the singer.

After some group experience, children can do the pantomiming individually. Give children with speech or listening problems a daily opportunity to practice their presentations of a particular record. It is helpful to have a mirror available so that they can watch their own interpretations.

Tell the children that good pantomiming to records involves constant movement of the whole body. There should be enough happening so that the viewer does not lose interest. I have found that humorous records are best for this experience. They seem to evoke the most response from the children.

Chapter Three

Creating Wholesome Environments

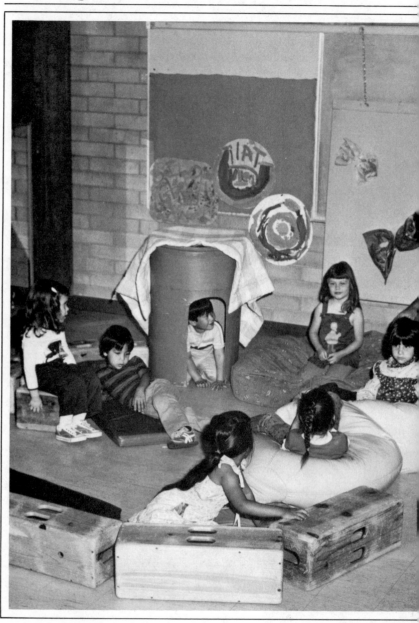

"Boys and girls. I have a surprise for you today. We're going to move all of the furniture out into the hallway and patio. Then, while I sit in the rocking chair having a nice quiet rest, you may fix up the room however you like and bring furniture back in and put it wherever you want to." Out went four tables, seventeen chairs, one bookcase full of books, one long toy cabinet full of manipulative toys, two block cabinets, several pieces of playhouse furniture, a record player, a portable closet full of dress-up clothes, mirrors, plants, science displays, and numerous other small items.

When we finished moving the furniture out, we all sat down on the floor in the newly empty room and had some apples and cheese. After the snack, I told the children to discuss with each other how they wanted to fix up the room.

The result was not at all what I expected. After careful consultation, the children brought in only three bean-bag pillows, three plastic-covered pillows, a barrel, and some hollow blocks. That was all.

For the next week the children had a fine time in their stripped-down room devoid of toy shelves and play equipment, books, records, and games. They rolled around on the floor, played games with each other, arranged and rearranged their meager furnishings, and basically enjoyed each other's company. What they had shown me was that, after several months of learning and socializing and growing in the carefully prepared environment I had arranged, their social skills had advanced to a point at which they were more interested in each other than in things. Because the room had been well-planned initially, it had helped, not interfered with, the children's growth.

Wholesome Environments

Restful and relaxing environmental settings can be creative, motivational, challenging, colorful, and educational. At the same time, they can present a casual atmosphere in which stressful situations are minimized, relaxation is an easy and natural part of the curriculum, and there is an underlying suggestion of serenity and tranquility.

Color, Light, Sound, and Climate

Color, lighting, acoustics, ventilation, air temperature, and humidity are all parts of the total environment. Give careful consideration to each. Walls should be painted restful, subdued tones; bright, intense colors can be overstimulating and create stress, while very dark colors can cause or reinforce gloomy, depressed feelings. I have done a number of experiments with color schemes in classrooms and have found blue-green combinations to be most soothing to young children.

Both too much light and too little light can raise levels of tension. Overstimulating the eyes with too much light causes fatigue; overworking the eyes because of too little light does the same. Fluorescent lights operate with a constant, subliminal flicker, that can be unconsciously irritating. Substitute incandescent lights for fluorescent lights whenever possible. Also be aware of glare from windows and from shiny surfaces—get down to the children's eye level to check—and do what you can to reduce it by using shades or curtains, painting table tops with matte finishes, and so forth.

Too much noise is a major cause of stress. Do what you can with drapes, carpeting, acoustical tile, and dropped ceilings to soften classroom noises and to keep outside noise from traffic and industry at a minimum. It might be useful to have a building inspector help you check the acoustics in the classroom.

Poor ventilation and too little humidity can cause headaches and upper-respiratory infections. Too much humidity and too hot a room can bring about feelings of lethargy. It's easy to see that it is important to achieve the right climate inside the class-room—not only for comfort, but for health and serenity as well. Check with a local utility company and ask if someone can help you evaluate your room's climate and can suggest methods for correcting inadequacies.

Bulletin Boards and Walls

The well-planned classroom has many play and work centers. Bulletin boards and other wall areas should complement these activity centers, rather than dominate the room. Children should be able to reach and touch the displays.

In preparing your learning environment for maximum rest-fulness, it's important to keep displays, decorations, and other movable objects at the children's eye level. In preschool class-rooms, don't place display items on bulletin boards, walls, or shelves any higher than 5 feet off the floor. For early primary grades, the height can go up to about 6 feet and still be com-fortable for the children. Remind yourself that children shouldn't have to strain their necks to look up at room decorations (in-cluding their own artwork). Another advantage of keeping every-thing low is that adults in the room will focus their eyes where the children are, instead of inadvertently being distracted by interest items above the children's heads.

Another consideration in planning room decorations is to leave some empty areas—*imagination space*. Sometimes walls are treated by teachers as though every bit of available blank space needs to have murals, children's work, posters, craft designs, pictures, you name it. If the walls are too busy, children won't be able to find a place for their eyes to rest, a blank slate for their imaginations to write on. Leaving room for imagination enhances the total philosophy of serenity in the classroom. A good working ratio for planning the use of wall space is one to two: one part of available wall space decorated with children's work and other displays, two parts left blank.

Equipment and Furnishings

Every teacher knows how important it is to have strong, stable, well-built equipment, furnishings, and playthings for the classroom. Flimsy, collapsing, easily breakable items can cause irritation to everybody using them. And constant admonitions to be careful and to watch out can be equally irritating. Stable, solid, well-crafted items will give the children a sense of security that will help them to feel safe and self-assured.

Unfortunately the costs of quality merchandise go up all the time. Rather than sacrifice quality, however, I suggest that you sacrifice quantity. Children can do just as well without many of the things that are found in classrooms. Most children like having a lot of open space as well as, or better than, having lots and lots of toys and equipment. Carefully choose the items that you do purchase. Solid wooden pieces give a feeling of warmth that is sometimes missing in plastic items. Be careful, however, that the wood you buy is really wood, and not some ersatz or camouflaged material made to look like wood. Obtain basic equipment and furnishings from a reputable educational supplier. If you can enlist the services of a talented carpenter, you may be able to design play pieces that will be at least equal to, and often superior to, those that you purchase.

In order to offset the expense of buying quality furnishings, you can supplement your room environment with many free or inexpensive materials. I make much use of heavy cardboard boxes which I get free of charge from appliance distributors and trash bins. I paint them with high-quality acrylic paint, which adds sturdiness to the boxes in addition to making them prettier.

Room Arrangements

Once you've planned and organized the setting, taking into account color, lighting, acoustics, durability, imagination space, and air and temperature control, you're ready to arrange the play and learning centers for maximum utility, motivation, and attractiveness. Remember, to create a casual, relaxed environment, room arrangements themselves ought to be casual and relaxed. The *central room arrangement plan* is a system I've devised to arrange the primary play–learning–study areas in the center of the room, with open areas on the periphery. The purpose of centralizing the individual activity centers is so that whenever children look up, they see and are near other persons instead of walls. This results in more natural conversation, more interaction between children of varied temperaments and interests, and a more relaxed and casual atmosphere. I have been challenged about this arrangement by some who say it works against achieving serenity in the classroom. Central arrangements do inspire children to be more talkative than if they were off in corners or along walls facing away from one another. But for normal, healthy, thinking children, talkativeness is a way of learning to use language meaningfully, of increasing social competence, and of developing interpersonal skills. The natural development of these abilities is central to inner serenity.

In the central room arrangement plan, the proximity of various types of centers encourages the fullest exploration of all the activities available. Children playing in such areas, or working on academic materials, do not feel isolated or pressured. Their backs are not vulnerable to unseen persons behind them. Yet they can also find many places to be alone outside the center of the room.

One of the primary functions of the central room arrangement plan is to allow for the flexible placement of play and learning centers. The orderly sameness of the room is maintained with bulletin boards, and very large pieces of furniture or equipment. The exact location of tables, chairs, and play materials can be slightly different from day to day. One week the housekeeping center might be right inside the entrance to the room, with the block area next to it, and tables with puzzles, art materials, and other play materials in the center of the room. The following week you might move the housekeeping corner to the opposite side of the room, put the blocks near the entrance, and have the painting area somewhere in between.

When there is a flexible room arrangement, children are encouraged to rearrange the placement and position of items to suit their own moods and inner feelings. Once invited to help arrange the room, children eagerly take part. They frequently discuss with their teachers ways in which they would like to see the room arranged. This involvement in room planning gives children a comfortable sense of belonging and acceptance, which leads to an overall reduction in emotional tension.

Easily Distracted Children

If you use the central room arrangement plan, you may find it necessary to have special places for easily distracted children to do tasks which require unusual amounts of concentration. These children should be placed facing a wall and away from other activities which involve much movement or talking. Hyperactive children function fairly well in the central room plan because their hyperactivity is not so obvious within the high-activity center area. When such children temporarily lose control, you can take them to a facing-the-wall work area. If you have two or three such children in a classroom, each can have a special enclosed space to be free to go to when isolation is needed.

The Dual-Purpose Room

When a room is used for play or other activities as well as for napping, the environment must be planned so that it will be conducive to sleep during the nap period.

If windows have pull-down blinds or another type of shade, the room can be darkened easily. Many classrooms, however, have large picture windows without drapes—and drapes are expensive (as is their upkeep). The best drapes are insulated, flameproofed, and as opaque as possible. Keep these facts in mind when ordering new drapes or replacing worn drapes.

If there are no shades or drapes for the windows, place cots so that the children's heads are away from the window side of the room. Move as many of the room furnishings as possible to one side of the room—leaving at least two walls completely bare to provide a clear view of the napping children and to increase the ease of leaving the room in case of fire.

Quiet Places

The activities throughout *Think of Something Quiet* are initiated and directed by adults. Children should be encouraged, however, to find their own times for quiet. The environment must provide comfortable places where children can isolate themselves from the distraction of others in the group, and where they can, temporarily, escape into their own peace and quiet. Such places should be attractive, cozy, and generally, just big enough for one child at a time. Pillows and small rugs of all kinds should be available to put in any of the quiet places for added comfort. Children's use of these places must be respected. They should have the freedom to use them when they feel the need, rather than when someone else tells them to. Emphasize that when a child is using an alone place, others may not intrude. The following suggestions are for quiet places that can be easily created in most classrooms.

◆§ The Alone Box

The alone box is an all-time favorite of teachers who use alone places. Obtain a cardboard box large enough for a child to lie down in or sit in comfortably on a small pillow. Washing machine, refrigerator, or stove cartons are satisfactory. You may be able to locate an equipment distributor who receives machinery packed in large boxes and is willing to save them for you.

Paint the box with a coat of good acrylic paint, and cut a small door in it. Place a large pillow or quilt on the floor and a sign reading "One Person Only" on the door.

◆§ The Barrel Box

Obtain a cardboard barrel that has contained some harmless substance such as flour, sugar, or other food item. Wash the barrel thoroughly and paint it with acrylics. Then cut an opening in one side. Place a soft, fluffy pillow in the barrel and a "One Person Only" sign on the outside.

✌§ Cloth Corners

You can make a quiet corner simply by stretching a makeshift canopy over an area and putting a pillow and a small rug on the floor. You can use decorative sheets or inexpensive yard goods; patterned materials are fine as long as the colors are subdued enough to enhance the relaxation process.

✌§ Behind-the-Furniture Places

Sometimes a quiet area, complete with rug, pillow, quilt, and two or three picture books can be arranged in a corner behind a piano, desk, or other large piece of furniture.

✌§ Rugs

A small section of an extra thick, luxurious carpet can provide enough of a contrast to the harder surface of the surrounding area that it immediately becomes a quiet place.

✌§ Sinking Places

Create "sinking" places with large bean-bag chairs or foam rubber chairs. You can make the bags from cloth that is soft and pleasant to touch, such as imitation fur. Fill the bags with small scraps of foam rubber or lightweight packing material. Place individual bags in unbusy corners, and let children sink into them to enjoy the tactile sensations and some quiet, cozy time.

✌§ Tent Places

Cover a table with a piece of material so that it drapes to the floor on all sides, and allow one child at a time to crawl under the table. The material should keep enough light out to create sufficient darkness to be calming, but let enough light in so that children won't become frightened at not being able to see where they are. Sheets and bedspreads make good coverings for tent places.

◆§ Wigwams

The tapering shape of either commercially manufactured or homemade wigwams is especially conducive to relaxation. It's a shape that seems to create a mood of gentle envelopment that provides a sense of being comforted and cared for.

◆§ Block Places

Children themselves can build private, alone places, with blocks of all kinds. I especially like cardboard brick blocks, which are very quiet when handled. These blocks are inexpensive enough so that you can have a great many available for children to use to construct their own private corners. Even marking out a private place with "walls" stacked one or two blocks high can give children the territorial satisfaction of having a place that only they are allowed to enter.

◆§ Tilted Tables

Tilting a table on its side and placing it in a corner is a simple way to make an alone place. The top and open ends can be closed off with pieces of cloth or throw rugs.

◆§ Benches

You can put two or more benches together for children to lie under. Place them along a wall, preferably in a corner, for maximum elimination of room light.

◆§ Chairs

Take three or four chairs, tilt them on their sides, and make a private place for someone who really feels the need to be alone. Such a place can be open or covered by a sheet or piece of cloth.

✒ Reading Table

Quiet places can be areas that have been arranged for reading for one or two children at a time. Use a small table next to a wall, placed so that the children using the table will see the wall when they look up, rather than the other activities in the room. The wall might have an interesting picture for the children to look at. The table should have an attractive cover, with several books neatly displayed to invite use.

✒ Library: No Talking

A bookshelf with three to four dozen carefully selected and nicely arranged books, a short room divider separating a small area from the rest of the room, and a comfortable fluffy rug on the floor can become a library. Talk with children about library rules: Books are to be put back neatly. Books may be shared with others, but aren't to be taken until the first reader is finished. Above all, no talking—only very, very quiet whispering. The library area should be limited to three or four children at a time.

✒ Drawing Table

A drawing table with large sheets of paper and a box of crayons creates an inviting quiet place. With room for only one child at a time, the table works best in a corner of the room or in a corner formed by the back of a piece of furniture and a wall. Two or three scribble-pictures on the wall will encourage children to use the crayons freely. Ten minutes of scribbling can do wonders to help an overexcited child calm down.

✒ Drawing Corner

Instead of the table, you can use a corner of the room by placing large sheets of paper on the floor. Encourage children to use all of the parts of the paper when drawing. Suggest that rather than crawling to the back of the paper to get to the other side, children can stretch way across the paper to reach the far corner. The purpose of such an activity is not the artwork, but the rhythmic use of crayons and body movements to bring children into a more relaxed state.

✒ Clay Place

Adults frequently overlook the therapeutic, calming effect on children of manipulating inexpensive plasticine. I recommend keeping a basket of plasticine, rolled into 2-inch balls, available and ready to bring out when children seem unduly tense and anxious. Some teachers keep a small table in an out-of-the-way corner stocked with plasticine balls. The children know that they are free to use this area whenever they want. Sometimes, too, angry or unhappy children might be encouraged to use the clay. After a few moments of rolling the clay between the hands to warm it up, the children begin to calm down—it's an acceptable, quiet manner to release accumulated nervous energy.

✒ Rainbow Corner

I like to use a rainbow or surprise corner as a place for children who appear to be depressed or unhappy, rather than tense or angry. Sometimes, just the specialness of using the surprise for the day will help a child relax and feel just a little more worthwhile. The rainbow corner can be permanent, in a quiet, out-of-the-way place, or it can involve the use of a prepared tray that a teacher brings out from time to time and places in a quiet corner. Items used should require minimum directions and can include the following:

1. Rainbows: A prism which can be picked up, examined, held up toward the light, and otherwise explored will provide myriad rainbows to enjoy.
2. Feathers: A box of feathers just to handle and explore can suggest soft, quiet movements.

3. Magnets: A group of magnets to attach to one another, or a horseshoe magnet and some iron filings or other metallic objects, can keep a child absorbed for some time.
4. Flannel board: A mini flannel board, with a variety of shapes for making designs, provides an eye-hand coordination exercise while encouraging relaxation.
5. One-color texture collage: Place on the table a small bottle of white glue, some pieces of paper of a single color, and a small container with a variety of objects to be glued. The more different textures you can get, the better. Try things like balloons, scraps of cloth, bits of plastic, string, ribbon, grasses, and flowers.

✒︎ Our Own Space

This activity helps children notice spatial relationships and gives them experience in deliberate isolation within a group. Suggest that children walk around the room and ask them to find a particular space that seems comfortable. Allow plenty of time. Suggest that they not get too close to other persons because they will need room for playing a game.

When all children have found suitable places, be certain they are all satisfied and comfortable, then proceed with the game. Pausing between suggestions, say:

In your space, feel the weight of your body on the floor. That space where your body is standing is your own space. No one else can be in that space. The floor in that little space is now part of you. Nice you. Nice floor. Sit down on the floor now. You need more floor space when you sit down. But it's still your space. Only you can be using that space right now. It really belongs to you. Feel the floor under you. Nice you. Nice floor.

Now, reach out with your hand, and draw a circle around your space. Make it whatever size you want without moving your body away from your space. Be sure you can reach all the sides of your circle with your arms while you're in the middle. As far as you can reach, that is your own space.

Touch the floor in your space. That's your very own floor. You can paint it a different color if you like. (Pretend to paint floor.) Or put a soft, fluffy carpet on it. You can put a big, bouncy mattress on it and jump up and down. Can you jump up and down in your space?

Maybe you would like to build a wall around your space. Well, just reach down to the floor like this (demonstrate) and build your wall as high as you want. You can build your wall high enough so that no one can see you inside. Be sure to build all the way around. Now you really have your own private place.

Perhaps you want to make a little window in your wall so you can see out. I'm going to make mine in the shape of a little heart. (Pretend to make window.) How are you going to make yours?

I think I'll paint my wall pink. I'm going to put fur on one side. Oh, I can lean against the fur and feel how soft it is. (Demonstrate.) What else can we do with our own space and the wall around it? We can make it stretchy. Push against it and stretch it way out, then let it bounce back in place again. (Demonstrate.) That feels good. Do it again.

Now I'm just going to be very quiet for a minute while you look around your own private space and decide what else you want to do to it. (Pause.)

How many of you like your space? I'm going to yell "Change!" When I do I want you all to run out of your own place and get into someone else's. "Change!" (Children all exchange places with one another.)

Is everyone in a new place? Do you like it as well as your own place? (The answer is generally "No!")

All right. "Change again!" You can all go back to your own places. How does that feel? Do you like it better than the new place you went to? You can all sit down and think about how it feels to have your very own place. (Pause for three or four minutes.) When you're ready, you can fold up your place and put it away. (Demonstrate.)

Chapter Four

Responding to Stress

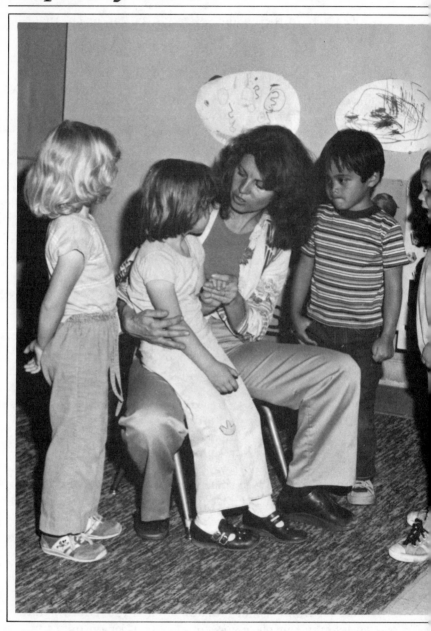

"O.K. I want everyone to settle down right now! Come back here. Put that down. No! Not that way! Over here. Come on. Pick it up. Careful. Oh, what a mess. Stop pulling her hair. Whoa! You may not throw those blocks. Ouch! That hurt me. That really hurt. Stop it right now. Stop fighting and play nicely with each other!"

This teacher, who is generally calm and good natured, was having a bad day. She was overtired and, for a moment or two, she really lost control of her emotions. The children had been playing vigorously for too long and she'd forgotten to take the usual midmorning break.

But now she paused, took a look around the room, pulled herself together, sat down, relaxed, and called the four quarreling children over to her. "Come on," she said. "Let's try to talk things over. We've all had such a busy morning, and I was letting myself get too tired. How about you?" There was an immediate camaraderie as the children realized that they were tired; they appreciated the fact that the teacher seemed to understand. She was even tired herself. They knew that she was going to help them feel better, and she knew that everything would soon be calm and serene again.

Signs of Fatigue

A normal group of children in an early childhood classroom will be active, talkative, and busy. Some children will enter the room and immediately start playing with others, some will choose to remain alone, and some will pair up with one special friend. Some will sit, some will stand, some will be in seemingly perpetual motion, and some will spend most of their time sitting on the floor.

As children play together, some will tire more easily than others. One of the first signs of physical tiredness is irritability. Another is anxiety. Tired children are frequently unduly sensitive and become emotionally distraught in social situations.

In your effort to maintain a calm and relaxing environment, it's important to be constantly alert to the signs of fatigue and stress in the children as they are going about their various activities. Often, by anticipating a deteriorating situation, you can offset the deterioration by gentle and thoughtful intervention.

It is important to become familiar with the signs of fatigue and stress. As you get to know each child's individual personality, you will adjust your judgment of a particular child's behavior accordingly. But there are some general warnings that you can watch for; they are outlined below.

VOICE SIGNALS
voice pitched higher than normal
voice much louder than usual
excessive and incessant talking
hoarseness
talking much faster than usual; words getting mixed up

APPEARANCE OF SKIN
flushed
pale
blotched

MOTOR CONTROL AND MOVEMENTS
stumbling and bumping into things
muscular tenseness

hyperactivity in an otherwise nonhyperactive child
inactivity in an otherwise active child; listlessness; dozing

EMOTIONAL TENOR
excitable
oversensitive; crying easily; quarreling
belligerent; angry

When you observe any of these symptoms, approach the child and try to determine if fatigue is the cause. Since some of these symptoms can also indicate the onset of an illness, one of the first things you might do is take the child's temperature to find out whether there is a fever. Learn what activities have preceded the symptoms. For example, any of the following activities could bring on fatigue, and possible stress:

- Vigorous physical exercise for an extended period of time (the length of time varies with the general physical condition and stamina of each child).
- An activity which may not be physically vigorous, but during which a child is exerting an unusual amount of mental effort.
- Any activity in which a number of children are involved. As with adults, groups can be tiring as one struggles to cope with the different personalities and moods of the individuals within the group.
- Any activity which a child is pursuing with extreme interest and concentration. Intense concentration is tiring to a young child after a time.
- Emotionally exciting experiences, such as birthday celebrations, intense musical activities, uninhibited laughing, rough-housing, and tickling. (Competitive games fall into this category. They are not recommended for children under five.)
- Sitting for too long in inactivity or being involved in a totally sedentary activity can cause mental fatigue.
- Noisy activities or a noisy environment is especially fatiguing to young children.

Offsetting a Fatiguing Activity

When you observe that children are showing signs of fatigue, you should intervene. The very fact that children are fatigued may prevent them from recognizing that they need to slow down, cease an activity, or rest.

The first step in intervention is planning. Does the curriculum accommodate both activities that require movement and physical effort and activities that are more sedentary? Does the classroom have quiet areas? If you take care to prepare the environment according to the suggestions given in this book, and if you have planned for alternating quiet and active experiences, you'll find it easier to guide children to a relieving change of pace when they are showing symptoms of fatigue.

The second step in intervention is prevention. Watch carefully for clues so that you can help children change their activity before fatigue overtakes them. When the first hint of fatigue appears, it is time to make a change. Don't wait until children are so tired that they lose emotional control.

Once you notice the onset of fatigue, give priority to helping children into relaxing situations. Sometimes this will mean spending time with one child alone, helping that child calm down sufficiently to be able to relax. You might say, "You're so flushed and out-of-breath. Come over here and rest a couple of minutes. I'll rub your arms a little. That always makes you feel better," or "Jennie, I'd like you to help me for a while. These balls of clay are too small. Will you try to roll them soft and then make two balls into one. Maybe that will be a better size. I'll help you." In another situation you might say, "You've been working hard with those blocks. That's sure going to be a nice building. I have an idea. I'll put a little sign that says, 'Keep Out,' and we'll ask everyone to leave the blocks alone. You can work on it again later, perhaps after lunch."

Often, relieving or preventing fatigue and stress will involve the entire group. Before doing any of the group activities included in *Think of Something Quiet*, you must consider what kind of physical arrangements will work best for the children.

Loose Arrangements

Throughout this book I have suggested that children sit on the floor in either a loose circle, a loose semicircle, or a loose formation (or free grouping). Loose arrangements maintain the semblance of a group, but allow each child to sit in a comfortable place and position. For example, I like to face the entrance to any room I'm in, no matter what the group structure. When I find myself with my back to the entrance, I keep adjusting my body to face the door. Some people prefer to sit behind others, while some like to be right in front. Many children are more comfortable sitting close to the teacher, while others feel better sitting away from the person in charge. In a semicircle, some children always want the apex position, while others prefer to sit elsewhere. Some prefer to face windows or lights, others, the opposite. When you allow for loose circling or grouping, all children can find comfortable places.

Anticipation for Quiet

To be certain a quieting, restful experience really is quieting and restful, you must anticipate that some children may cause a disturbance if they are sitting next to best friends or to someone whom they dislike. Two aggressive children, or two giggly friends, or other disruptive combinations, can be handled in advance by a kind of gentle interference I call *teaching by anticipation*. Matter-of-factly say, "Jeremy, I would like you to trade places with Stephanie," or "Jeremy, I want you to sit there between Stephanie and Suzette." I try to direct a noisy, restless, or aggressive child to sit between two mild-mannered, quiet ones. In moving Jeremy, however, remember to be aware of his comfort. You might end up rearranging several children in order to separate Jeremy from his friend, but at the same time, maintain his right to be as comfortable in his position as are the others. As long as a loose structure is maintained from the beginning, children can usually tolerate my anticipatory interference.

To Stand or to Sit

Although many of the activities in *Think of Something Quiet* rec-ommend standing, sitting in a chair, or sitting on the floor, these are only suggestions. Children can do the activities in many different situations and positions. Feel free to make changes and adaptations that make you more comfortable. If you are com-fortable and at ease, the children are more likely to be comfort-able and at ease.

When children sit in chairs, their feet should rest solidly on the floor. Be sure children don't sit on their feet when sitting on the floor; sitting that way can cause foot deformities in very young children. Instead they should sit either cross-legged or with their legs stretched out in front of them.

When resting at tables or desks using the arms as cushions, children should rest their heads against the backs of the hands, rather than the forearms. The weight of the head on the forearms can slow down the natural flow of blood and can cause the arms to grow numb.

Muscular Exercise for Relaxation

Muscular overexertion can cause so much tiredness and muscular tension that relaxation becomes difficult. However, muscular ex-ercise, used in moderation, can have the opposite effect and can aid in relaxation.

When children have been playing vigorously, running hard and long, climbing, jumping, and otherwise using their muscles to the point of exhaustion, they frequently will come to a sudden halt and flop themselves down on the ground, breathless. At such times, it is best to try to slow them down gradually. Have children lie on their backs, and suggest the following activities.

❧ Angels in the Snow

Have children start with their bodies held straight, legs together, arms touching sides. When you say "open," legs spread wide apart and arms reach up behind heads, keeping as much of the body as possible in contact with the floor. When you say "close," limbs go back to the starting position. The count should be slow, becoming slower and slower as the game progresses.

This is an integrative exercise that is relaxing because it requires equal control of all four limbs at one time. Also, the sensation of the surface against legs and arms extends the tactile, rhythmic effect equally throughout the body, increasing the ability of all parts of the body to function harmoniously.

After they slow down somewhat, children can do some of the breathing exercises described on pages 92–96.

Exercise After Sedentary Periods

Sometimes too long a period of inactivity, or too long a period of sitting in one position, can cause the body to feel too tense for comfort.

✍ Sitting-up Exercises

Gentle sitting-up exercises are an aid to the general loosening of stiff muscles and to stimulation of the flow of oxygen throughout the bloodstream. If these exercises are used to aid relaxation, take care to avoid letting them become too strenuous. They should be done very slowly, in a standing position.

Arms up over the head, straight out to the sides, down at the sides.

Arms straight out in front, out to the sides, down at the sides.

Arms straight out in front, up over the head, down at the sides.

Arms straight out to the sides, out in the front (clapping hands together), down at the sides.

Legs apart, arms out to the sides, hands touching the floor, stand up straight again.

Arms over the head, hands touching the toes, stand up straight again.

Knees straight, knees bent, knees straight again.

Knees straight, arms out to the sides, knees bent, knees straight, arms down at the sides.

Legs apart, left hand touching right toe, stand up straight again.

Legs apart, right hand touching left toe, stand up straight again.

Continue with similar exercises, limiting each to three or four. repetitions.

Relaxation of Tension through Humor

Sometimes we get so caught up in our adult roles that we forget about the power (and gentleness) of humor. One stormy day when the children couldn't play outside, the walls seemed to be closing in, and tension was building, I suddenly went to a cupboard, opened the door, and shouted.

"Come out of there. Come out of there right now. You know people aren't allowed in there. You come out right now."

The room was still as all eyes focused on the cupboard.

I reached my hand inside and continued, "Well, I'll just have to take you out. Now hold still. Now I've got you. No! Hold still, will you. Ah, hah! I have you."

Out came my hand, fist rolled up, with a simple smiling face drawn on it.

I continued the conversation by scolding the face for smiling when it had made me so angry. "Why do you keep smiling at me like that? Don't you know we have a rule: No one plays inside the cupboard. Now stop that. Stop smiling at me."

By then, all of the children had joined in, and we decided to sing a song about smiles.

Another tense day, wanting to lower the noise level that was building up, I opened the outside door and said, to an invisible being, "Why good morning, Nothing. Please come in."

Some nearby children stopped what they were doing to watch me.

"Won't you please sit down, Nothing," I said as I pulled a chair out from a table and placed it near the center of the room.

By now, the rest of the children had stopped what they were doing to watch me. Jessica said, "But there's nobody."

I said, "That's why I called the person Nothing. Jessica, you may go to the door and invite someone in."

Jessica brought another Nothing in. So did Tommy. Now we had three chairs lined up. Barbara was next. She invited in Mr. Invisible. This started their imaginations working. Stuart asked But-I-Can't-See-You to come in and sit down. Maria opened the door for Mrs. Zero, and Louise invited George the Ghost in.

The game continued until all children had opened the door for invisible beings and had set out chairs for them. Then I said, "Now, everybody sit on your friend's lap."

As the children scrambled to the chairs of their guests, there was a relaxed atmosphere of fun and camaraderie that had come from sharing this silliness with the teacher.

While considering silliness games, remember to include some silly songs in your children's music repertoire.

THE BEAR WENT OVER BANANA
(Tune: "The Bear Went Over the Mountain")

The bear went over banana,
The bear went over banana,
The bear went over banana,
To see what it could eat.

The gooshy part of banana,
The gooshy part of banana,
The gooshy part of banana,
Was all that it could eat.

The bear went into the oven.
The bear went into the oven,
The bear went into the oven
To see what made it hot.

The bear came out of the oven,
The bear came out of the oven,
The bear came out of the oven,
And hot was all it got.

The child who made this last verse was an instant hero, as everyone joined in the laughter and repeated over and over the last line, "And hot was all it got."

This tension-releasing activity was especially effective because we were totally involved with one another in enjoying the silly humor. Following such a tension-releasing experience, it is very easy to say to the children: "Boys and girls, look at me." (Pause.) "Now, I want everyone to think of something quiet."

However, it is also an appropriate time to simply say, "Let's all lie down for a few moments and just listen to our own quiet."

Emergency!

There are times when children are so out of control that you need to take emergency measures before you can begin to think about using relaxation techniques. The follow examples illustrate some things that work in times of emergency.

STROKING
Gently stroking a child's back or arms or shoulders will help ease tense muscles. Stroking can have a fairly rapid therapeutic effect on a tense, overtired child.

HOLDING
Approaching a child from behind and wrapping your arms tightly about her or him will sometimes help to calm a tantrum.

HUGGING
Hugging is especially helpful for drying tears. Hugging with a rocking motion can be soothing to jangled nerves.

ISOLATION
Being alone in a comfortable space, without nagging or quizzing, can give an out-of-control child an opportunity for some much-

needed emotional release. Children need reassurance during such times that it is all right for them to be upset and to express their feelings in their own way. It is better to let children release their emotions than to suppress them. Isolation means that there is no audience for tantrums, crying jags, or emotional outbursts, but that someone is near to give physical comfort and reassurance when it's all over.

ENCOURAGEMENT
There are some children who get so out of control that you must help them regain control to keep them from getting too physically exhausted. One technique that works with some children is to encourage them to cry louder, to scream harder, to kick something (unbreakable!), to stamp on the floor, or to bang fists on a table top. Just stopping to respond to the suggestion is a change of pace. If I see that children have paused even for an instant to hear what I am saying, then I know that they are no longer out of control.

FOOD
A nutritional snack, unless the child is too agitated to eat, will sometimes speed the relaxation of tense muscles.

Comfort for Life Crises

To help children achieve the serenity that is their right, we must learn to be aware of their home and family lives as well as their interactions with others at school. Much that happens at home that can seem ordinary to adults can be the source of the anxiety and stress that you see in the classroom. Family problems and situations may cause anything from mild concern to severe trauma in children. A child might not even be directly involved—it may be something happening to a relative or friend or even a casual acquaintance of the family. Fear, ignorance of the true nature of a situation, and imagination, can combine to create a serious emotional crisis in the child. Some situations that can create these crises are:

- An illness, pain, or hospitalization of child, friend, or relative.
- A visit to a doctor or dentist.
- A new baby in the home.
- An older sibling leaving home for work, college, marriage, or just a temporary trip.
- A parent leaving the home temporarily for a vacation, business trip, or other reason.
- A parent leaving because of separation or divorce.
- A move to a new home.
- Another child or adult moving into a child's own home.
- Adoption by another family.
- Parents' financial problems.
- Parents' work and social schedules.
- An older sibling in trouble at school.
- A parent or relative in trouble with the law.
- A death or a terminal illness.
- Loss of a pet through illness, accident, or runaway.
- A natural disaster such as an earthquake, flood, hurricane, tornado.
- Extremes of weather such as strong winds, rain, snow, fog, thunder, and lightning.
- Preparing to go on a family trip or vacation.
- Forest fires nearby; home fires.
- Actions of a drunken parent, relative, or friend.
- The presence of strangers in the home.

Sometimes just small things have conditioned children to develop certain fears. An affectionate dog may have licked an infant on the face, so frightening the child that years afterward dogs or other small animals still produce an automatic fear reaction.

Don't overlook the fears and misunderstandings that can arise from watching adult-oriented television shows, commercials, and movies. I once experienced a situation in which a four-year-old girl sobbed and cried bitterly for almost two hours. She bore no sign of physical hurt. She wouldn't answer my questions. Finally, I had won her trust enough for her to say, between sobs,

"My brother told me I had ba-aa-d breath." This was at a time when one frequently shown commercial depicted some very ugly, distorted faces as having bad breath. The child was identifying herself with the ugliness in the ad.

Unthinking adults can create fears and tension in children by setting standards for achievement too high, by being extremely harsh with discipline, and by frequently ridiculing and criticizing children. Unfortunately, it is not always easy to get children to talk about the reasons behind their behavior. It becomes your task to put together the observable symptoms, the situations, and the incidents you are aware of, and then to evaluate them in relation to the individual child's personality and physical and emotional characteristics.

It's always helpful to hear from home about unusual circumstances that may cause the child to act differently from usual. To encourage such communication, I send home a letter, similar to the one following, two or three times each year.

Dear Parents,

Children are extremely vulnerable to their environment and to people in their lives to whom they feel close. Sometimes things happen at home, especially among the adult members of the family, that may disturb or confuse children. Perhaps there was a quarrel, a discussion of financial difficulties, an illness, or unexpected visitors. These things might create tension—tension to which children react.

Tension-creating incidents are not necessarily unpleas-ones. Perhaps someone is planning a trip, or the family is making plans for welcoming visitors, or new furniture is arriving, or the carpenter is coming to make some alterations. Perhaps there are preparations for a big dinner party. These things may cause children to be emotionally keyed up and may cause them to react more quickly and negatively to otherwise normal incidents. It may be that the tension-creating incident was a very minor thing to you—missing car keys, a rush to make a 9:00 A.M. appointment, the toast burned three times in a row. You even might have exclaimed over the latest newspaper headlines or complained because the newspaper wasn't even delivered.

Whatever the incident, you may have unwittingly imparted unusual feelings of tension to your child. You may have dealt with your own tensions by being short-tempered, overly stern, or even by spanking.

It might not have been anything anyone else did at all. Children can become upset (just as we sometimes do) over the color of the only clean shirt there is to wear or a hole in a favorite pair of socks. It is difficult enough to understand the workings of someone else's mind—but it is especially difficult to understand the minds of children. We do know, however, that their feelings, tensions, and emotions are real.

We are striving to promote an underlying atmosphere of serenity throughout our school. You can help us.

If you notice that your child seems unusually tense, or if you know there was indeed an unpleasant or stressful situation in the home, please let us know. We prefer that you don't talk about it in front of your child. You can write a brief note, call us by phone, or talk to us privately at school. Needless to say, the information you give us will remain strictly confidential.

We will try to use all information to understand your child's needs, to help restore lost composure, and to calm anxieties. We will appreciate all the help you can give us in trying to make each new school day an exciting, fulfilling, joyful experience for your child. It is our goal to send your child home each day feeling relaxed and fulfilled. Please know that we are eager to be of assistance in whatever way is needed.

Very sincerely,

Abused and Deprived Children

Unfortunately, a letter will have little or no effect on the parents of children who come from very deprived or abusive environments. These children may show signs of tension through such actions as nail-biting, fidgeting, being easily irritated or upset, crying or silently sobbing, or fighting. On the other hand, many of these children are very passive and quiet. They have retreated into themselves and have built protective facades.

If you suspect a child is being abused, or if you witness abuse, follow through. If abuse is verbal, discuss with parents the fact that their manner of speaking to children is a kind of abuse; this may be of some help. Physical abuse should be reported to the appropriate local authorities. Potentially abusive parents can be referred to a Parents Anonymous or a similar group, existing in many communities. Local mental health groups can provide the needed information about organizations that will give the parents the help they seek.

Meanwhile, you have the abused or deprived children in your care much of the day. These children respond well to constant reassurance that you are aware of their presence and that you are pleased with it. They should be spoken to a great deal in soft, gentle, reassuring tones and words. Though at first they may pull back from your direct touch, don't give up — they need a great deal of physical comfort and caressing. Teaching them some of the techniques of mind and body relaxation presented in *Think of Something Quiet* may help them toward achieving some semblance of balance and serenity within their troubled selves.

Books

There are many books, written especially for children, that can be helpful in facing various life crises and traumas and in overcoming fears. Nothing can replace the comfort that comes from being touched, hugged, held, stroked, and sincerely cared for. But sometimes even the most empathetic response still doesn't solve the puzzlement and confusion. A story, or an illustrated book, can frequently bridge that gap between human caring and childhood misunderstanding.

Don't expect the books to provide all the answers. You'll need to follow up with discussions, questions, answers, and even, at times, some role-playing. The best books are usually the simplest ones. Length is not the criterion. Rather, look for relevance to the issue or problem, reasonable illustrations with which children can identify, and language that is honest and forthright, but on a child's level. The Bibliography at the end of this book lists several children's books dealing with various life crises.

The Weather

Young children can be very confused by changing weather conditions. Extremes of weather can cause tensions which should not be ignored. Helping children to understand the changing seasons and the surprises of the weather can help ease their tensions regarding it.

◄§ Weather Game

To help children feel more comfortable with various kinds of weather, play this game which has them act out what they'd do in many different weather situations. Say:

> Pretend you are. . .
> walking in the rain
> playing in the sandpile on a very hot day
> walking barefoot on a hot sidewalk
> playing in the snow
> walking through very deep snow
> walking through a fog
> walking through puddles left by the rain
> carrying an opened umbrella to keep off the rain
> sharing an umbrella with someone else (two children do
>   this together)

getting caught in the rain without a raincoat; getting soak-
   ing, dripping wet
rolling down a snow-covered hill
wiping the steam off of the windows to see out
wearing so many clothes that you can hardly move when
   you go outdoors to play
deciding to stay in bed and keeping warm under your covers
   while it's lightning and thundering outdoors
trying to walk while a very strong wind is blowing against
   you
trying to walk while a very strong wind is blowing behind
   you

Windy Days

Windy days may be confusing, sometimes frightening, to young
children. The abnormal amount of electricity in the air causes
all of us to become more tense than usual. Tempers may be short,
nerves may be taut, and children may have difficulty in retaining
their composure if the adults around them aren't calm.

   On windy days it can be helpful to discuss the weather,
particularly what the wind does and what causes it to blow. Talk
about air and air movement, and explore the nature of wind.
The following simple experiences will help children to understand the qualities and function of wind:

* Look outdoors. How many things can you see that are
  being blown by the wind?
* Pretend being the wind. Make a small wind by blowing
  with your mouth.
* Take something heavy and something light outdoors, and
  see which blows away the quickest.
* Take something wet outdoors. Put a similar wet object
  indoors. See whether it dries faster outside in the wind
  or indoors.
* Observe the movement of clouds, if any.
* Make wind-blowers as follows: Cut strips of crepe paper

into 6-foot lengths. Tie several strips together around the middle, using a 2-foot length of yarn made into a loop. Holding the loop, allow the crepe paper to blow in the wind. Run while holding the loop. Does the crepe paper blow differently?

• Sing "The Wind Is Blowing All Around" found below; while singing, ask children to pretend that they are the wind.

• Pretend to be tall trees in the wind. Sing "The Tall Trees," shown below.

THE WIND IS BLOWING ALL AROUND
(Tune: "Mary Had a Little Lamb")

The wind is blowing all around, all around, all around,
The wind is blowing all around, all around the air.
The leaves are shaking in the trees, in the trees, in the trees,
The leaves are shaking in the trees, and make a rustling
    sound.

THE TALL TREES
(Tune: "Frère Jacques")

Tall trees standing, tall trees standing,
    On the hill, on the hill,
See them all together, see them all together,
    So very still. So very still.
Wind is blowing, wind is blowing,
    On the trees, on the trees,
See them swaying gently, see them swaying gently,
    In the breeze. In the breeze.
Sun is shining, sun is shining,
    On the leaves, on the trees,
Now they all are warmer, and they all are smiling,
    In the breeze. In the breeze.

Activities for windy days should be kept as low-key as possible. Take every opportunity to play touching games and to be close together as a group.

Foggy Days

Foggy days can also be frightening to young children who may not have experienced many such days. Their usual vision is obscured, yet they know it isn't night. Riding in automobiles, they hear the drivers express despair, and perhaps even fear about not being able to see the road and other cars clearly. These expressions of real concern can make children feel uneasy and tense. You can initiate a variety of activities to ease their tensions in such situations:

- Talk about clouds that children have seen up in the sky, and suggest that the fog is a cloud that is resting on the ground.
- Greet children, upon arrival, with such comments as, "I'm glad you're here. It must have been hard riding through the fog," or "It must have been hard to see where the car was going. I'm glad you arrived safe and sound."
- Boil some water to produce steam. Allow the steam to fog a mirror or window.
- Make fog by blowing breath outdoors.
- Paint with black and white paint (on white paper) to make foggy clouds.

Stormy Days

Stormy days, too, can be upsetting to young children. The first day or two of stormy weather may be exciting because children get to wear raincoats and boots. Unfortunately, however, adults often become irritable after two or three consecutive days of rain. This irritation affects children, and as children become irritable, the adults around them usually become more so.

You can survive stormy weather by using a number of techniques, such as:

- Talk about stormy weather. Talk about what kinds of feelings stormy weather causes. Why? Encourage children to talk about being scared of lightning, thunder, and heavy downpours.

- Read stories about stormy weather situations. Children's librarians will help you find many books about sailing ships that had to weather storms, about islands and subtropical parts of the world where it rains often, and other related topics.
- Make rain pictures. Tape paper on windows or easels. Mix tempera paint so that it is fairly thin. Use the largest paintbrushes you have. Demonstrate how, if the brush is pressed against the paper, the paint will drip down the paper, making "colored rain." Vary the colors from day to day to extend the project during a long rainy spell.
- Discuss the benefits of rain: It provides us with drinking water, water to use in the house, and water to make things grow.
- Play a game in which children curl themselves up as small as they can and pretend to be seeds planted in the ground. Have them feel the rain come down on them. The seeds swell when they drink the rainwater. (Children slowly uncurl themselves.) They get ready to grow into big vegetables and flowers and trees. (Children sprout up off the floor.)
- Have the children be raindrops running all over the room. Raindrops start out so quietly, on tiptoes; then they get louder and faster until finally, spent, they slow down again to a soft, gentle shower.
- Do a weather play, similar to the following, substituting the types of weather phenomena that are taking place in your locale. (As you tell the story, various children can act out particular roles which are preassigned, or the entire group can act out each role as it comes along.)

I WOKE UP ONE MORNING

I woke up one morning and looked out the window. It was raining gently. All of the raindrops (children) were playing tag all over the yard and the sidewalk and everywhere I looked. Suddenly I heard loud thunder (children make loud thunder). A minute later there was a big flash of lightning going from one side of the world to the other (children run like lightning from one side of the room to the other). Then it began to rain very hard. Big loud drops just poured and poured and poured out of the sky (children jump up and down mimicking heavy rain). It rained so much that all of the kitty cats hid in corners. (Children hide in corners like kitty cats.) The trees spread out their branches and stretched their roots and drank all of the water they could (children become trees). The water made them strong and straight and healthy. There was more thunder! (Pause.) More lightning! (Pause.) And then it hailed (if there is hail in your area). The hail made noise when it hit the buildings. Pretty soon, just as I watched, everything became quiet. The rain had changed to snow (children become snow). The snow was so quiet as it fell to the earth that it made the world feel as if it had a nice, comfortable, warm blanket over it. When all of the snow lay covering the ground, I went to my room to get dressed and ready for school.

Chapter Five

Getting the Most from Rest Times

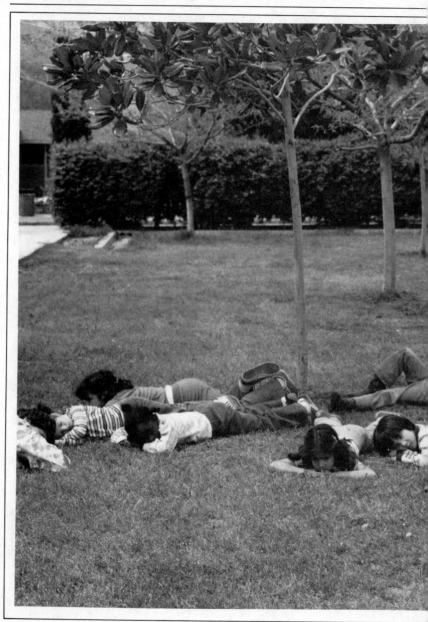

It was an unusually lively, joyful day. The children were decorating their rooms in preparation for a family supper that was to be held that night. Routines were changed, furniture was moved around, and there was a great deal of laughing and playful repartee. At a certain point, I realized that a few of the children were becoming tense and quarrelsome. I knew that they had to be taken to a quieter place to calm down and to rest for a while. Everything was so busy indoors that I decided to find a place outside. I stood at the door leading to the patio and began to chant, slowly and quietly:

Softly on his tip-tip toes,
The animal through the forest
    goes.
Lion, tiger, caribou,
Deer, giraffe, and zebra, too.
Shhh! Shhh! Shhh!

When the children joined me we walked quietly out to the lawn as I repeated the chant. We stopped at the newly planted magnolia tree. I said that the shiny green leaves were asking us to lie down and rest awhile. We all found a comfortable position on the lawn and basked in the sun.

Resting Is Not Just a "Break"

Young children respond best to programs that have alternating rhythms of active play and quiet experiences. The adults in such programs know that it is frequently necessary to have one or two particular children, or an entire group of children, rest for brief periods to prevent them from becoming overstimulated and overtired. These adults often find it difficult to quiet children who have been playing busily and vigorously, especially if there has been a high degree of tension in the atmosphere. When the children finally do rest, all too often it is considered to be merely a chance for the adult to rest.

It is important to ask yourself, "What does the rest period do for the children?" You may never have considered it more than a chance for children to quiet down. You may have felt that all the children need to do is just rest.

Just resting isn't enough. Although resting may help to offset physical and mental fatigue, it is of minimal benefit to the physical and emotional growth of the children unless they can be wholly relaxed and totally involved with the experience.

The adult facilitator is the key to the children's total involvement. If you allow yourself to become completely immersed in a resting mood and spirit, you will transmit to the children a feeling that will help them get the most from the experience. Avoid being brisk and hurried. Establish a mood of tranquility by your own gentle movements, your hushed voice, and your pleasant demeanor. Dim the lights and walk softly. Let the children know that you are feeling a little tired and that it will make you feel better to have a chance to rest with them for a while. Above all, don't think of this as a time to escape. What you once looked upon as just a necessary, routine part of your job can become one of the most pleasurable and meaningful parts of the total day.

Short Resting Times

When short rest periods are part of a morning or afternoon class session or an after-nap playtime, it isn't necessary to depend on cots. In fact, children who resist rest periods of any kind may be more cooperative when they are not asked to use equipment that is normally used for napping.

It is helpful always to give children a few moments of warning before the rest period, saying, "In a few minutes I'll want you to stop what you're doing so we can all take a short rest."

Resting times can be preceded or followed by any of the relaxation exercises in *Think of Something Quiet.* However you proceed, remember that young children appreciate routines; routines lend security and comfort to a world which is constantly presenting them with new challenges and new ideas. Children participating in spontaneous, brief resting periods, routinely performed in the same way, learn to relax at will. As their ability to do so increases, they are more likely to develop a deeper appreciation of their inner selves and the human striving for tranquility.

Begin all rest periods with breathing exercises. Stop the vigorous play that may have become overstimulating, and call the children to gather around you. Suggest that everyone take a deep breath (following your own example) and exhale slowly. Repeat the exercise four or five times. (See page 92.)

Remember to anticipate potential commotion when making resting arrangements. Separate giggly pals and intersperse aggressive and boisterous children among calm ones.

Children can sit at tables for a few moments' rest. They make a cushion by cradling their arms together and overlapping their hands. They put their heads down on the cushion their hands make and close their eyes. Help the children place their arms in such a way that they actually put their heads down on their hands. Pressure on the arms can slow down blood circulation and upset the natural flow of oxygen in the bloodstream. To avoid the problems that arise when children stare into each other's eyes and giggle and whisper, suggest that everyone face in the same direction. Be sure that the position is comfortable for each child. If not, it is better to make an exception than to defeat the entire purpose by causing undue tension.

Sometimes you can create a good, abbreviated rest period simply by having all of the children lie down on their backs. This is an especially good resting position to use outdoors, when children can look up at the sky as they relax and watch clouds. If the room has a large carpeted area, children can lie on the floor, cradling their arms. If there is no large carpeted area children can use individual rugs or commercially produced resting mats. I like to use the woven rag rugs that are commonly sold in variety stores for use in kitchens. They wash easily, are comfortable to lie on, and are long-wearing. They are generally available in small (2½ by 3 feet) and medium (2½ by 4 feet) sizes, which I find adequate for children from ages two through eight. Even the youngest children can learn to fold them and place them in their appropriate storage area when they are through resting.

Children might have their own pillows to use at resting time. They should be about 3 or 4 inches thick. Too thick a pillow can be harmful to postural development. Too thin a pillow doesn't cushion well enough. Each pillow should have the owner's name attached. Whether brought from home or provided by the school, the pillows should have washable covers which are periodically laundered.

Storytelling and Other Activities

Some stories have cues that help the listener to concentrate and to relax. If you have two or three such stories, and if you present them in a quiet, easy manner, the stories themselves will become the cues for relaxation after they have been used several times. Repetition is comfortable to young children. They like to know what's going to happen next. They like to know in advance that the crisis will be solved and that the story will have a happy ending.

I like to tell stories while sitting on the floor (or on the ground, if outdoors), with the children gathered close around me so my voice can be dramatized, yet soft. I like to encourage the children to keep their hands on their knees while listening to the stories. They respond well to my gentle reminders, since I am consistent and use this technique every time. You may find it difficult at the beginning. Just keep interrupting your story and giving reminders such as, "Where are your hands, Sara?" or "Bobby, are your hands on your knees?" Soon you will discover that everyone is sitting more quietly and more relaxed. Without the distractions of poking, pulling, punching, scratching, and picking, attention remains focused and story time can be a truly magical time.

It's very important that you enjoy the stories you tell. Your own enjoyment will bring you closer to the listeners.

✍ Tell an Eyes-Closed Story

Eyes-closed stories are told when children are actually resting while sitting at tables with their heads down, or lying down. Tell the story very, very slowly and in as quiet a voice as possible, almost a whisper, just loud enough for all children to hear.

Eyes-closed stories should have special sounds as cues for which the children listen. The stories are heavy with imagery and environmental suggestions which are conducive to rest and relaxation. They use much repetition, almost hypnotic in effect, but have occasional changes in pace to maintain interest. One story that I have used hundreds of times follows. It is one that I still enjoy telling just as much as the children enjoy listening to it. An advantage of this kind of story is that it can be shortened or lengthened to fit available time. To shorten the story, simply leave out some of the animals and skip to the birds near the end of the story. To lengthen the time, add some animals of your own.

AND EVERYONE WAS SOUND ASLEEP

It was getting dark outside.

"Oh-ho," I said. "It's time to go to sleep."
I made a little pillow with my arms and put my head down on my cushiony hands just like this (demonstrate). I closed my eyes, and listened to the quiet, quiet world.
(Pause for children to get comfortable and to close their eyes. Remind them that this is an eyes-closed story.)
At first I didn't hear anything at all. But I was very

quiet, and I listened very hard. Soon I heard a tiny, squeaky sound saying, "Meow. Meow. Meow." I knew what that was. That was my baby kitty cat saying, "Goodnight. Goodnight. Goodnight." Then my kitty cat rolled itself into a furry ball, put its head down on its paws just like you, and soon was sound asleep.

The world was very quiet.
The house was very quiet.
I was very quiet, and I listened very carefully.
Soon I heard another sound. It went, in a tiny, tiny voice, "Woof-woof. Woof-woof. Woof-woof." That was the little puppy dog who lived next door, saying, "Goodnight. Goodnight. Goodnight." Then the puppy dog put its head down on its paws, just like the kitty cat and just like you. It closed its eyes and soon was sound asleep.

The world was very quiet.
The house was very quiet.
I was very quiet, and I listened very carefully.
Soon I heard the little calf who lived down at the corner with the farmer. The calf, in its little baby voice, said, "Moo-moo. Moo-moo. Moo-moo. Goodnight. Goodnight. Goodnight." And soon the calf was sound asleep. Then the baby pig said, "Oink-oink. Oink-oink. Oink-oink. Goodnight. Goodnight. Goodnight." And the baby pig put its head down, just like the kitty cat and the puppy dog and you. And soon it was sound asleep. Then I heard the baby horse say, "Neigh. Neigh. Neigh. Goodnight. Goodnight. Goodnight." It closed its eyes just like you and soon was sound asleep. And all of the farm animals who lived with the farmer were very quiet.

The world was very quiet.
The house was very quiet.
I was very quiet, and I listened very hard.
I didn't hear a thing.
Far, far away across the ocean, over the fields at the bend of the river, in the jungles where all the wild animals lived, the baby tiger was getting sleepy, too. The baby tiger wanted to say goodnight to its mommy and daddy, so it opened its mouth very wide and said (in a

tiny voice), "Roar. Roar. Roar." It was just a very tiny roar because it was just a very tiny baby tiger. It was saying, "Goodnight. Goodnight. Goodnight." It put its head down on its paws, closed its eyes just like you, and soon was sound asleep.

Next door to where the tigers lived, a baby giraffe stretched its long giraffety neck and didn't make a sound. Giraffes don't know how to make noise. But it kissed its mommy and daddy goodnight, sat down on the ground with its long neck sticking right up in the air, closed its eyes, and soon was sound asleep.

The world was very quiet.

And there, across the ocean, over the fields at the bend of the river, in the jungles where all the wild animals lived, everyone was sound asleep.

The house was very quiet.

I was very quiet, and I listened very carefully. (Pause. Use slight change of pace.)

Suddenly, up in the treetops, the baby birds began to sing. "TWEET! TWEET! TWEET!" They were not being quiet at all. Mama bird began to scold them and she said, "Shhh! Shhh! Shhh!" The baby birds said very quietly, "Tweet. Tweet. Tweet. Goodnight. Goodnight. Goodnight." They tucked their heads under their wings, closed their eyes just like you, and soon they were all sound asleep.

And not a twitter or a tweet was heard in all the wide, wide world.

One by one the stars began to shine.

There was a star for _____, and a star for _____ (continue as you name each resting child, giving a gentle pat on the head as each name is mentioned).

The moon came out and saw all of the children sleeping. It smiled its biggest smile and sang this lullaby (or say, ". . . played this music"). (Sing lullaby or play record.) (Wait.) (Continue in a cheerful tone of voice.) Then the sun came out, the lights came on, and everyone sat up and said, "Hello."

(Quiet time is over.)

◄§ Arm Movement Game

Movements of the arms, which include shoulder movements, are conducive to the release of tension. Many of the activities throughout this book incorporate arm movements. The following game is specifically devoted just to arm movements. Even older elementary-aged children enjoy this game. It gives them a chance to role-play, while it encourages relaxation. To play it, have the children lie on their backs with their bodies straight.

BABY, BABY, IN YOUR BED
(Tune: "Twinkle, Twinkle, Little Star")

Baby, baby, in your bed,
You cannot lift your tired head,
But you can reach your arms way out,
Reach and stretch them all about,
Reach your arms way up so high,
Reach and stretch them to the sky.

Baby, baby, in your bed,
You cannot lift your tired head,
But you can reach your legs way out,
Reach and stretch them all about,
Reach your legs way up so high,
Reach and stretch them to the sky.

As you repeat the song, soften your voice so that children can barely hear you, and say, "If you listen very hard, you can probably hear the inside of you move."

◄§ Finger Games

Traditionally, teachers use finger games during transition periods and quiet times. You don't need to have a large repertoire. (See the Bibliography at the end of the book for titles of finger-game books.) Children love the repetition of a few favorites. Hearing the same ones over and over again makes it easy for them to follow along without stress. The repetition itself is relaxing. Don't try to do too many, but vary them from time to time.

• Use children's names. For example, in singing "Teensy

weensy spider goes up the water spout," you could say: "Teensy weensy Barbara goes up the water spout. . . ."
- Vary the tone of your voice. Select a favorite game that all of the children know. First use your normal voice. Then repeat it in a high, squeaky voice. The third time do it in a low, gruff voice. Another way to vary the tone is to repeat the game over and over, saying it just a little more quietly each time until finally you are doing only the motions and not the words.
- Say all of the lines to a finger-game rhyme, such as Time to Rest on this page. Repeat the rhyme, leaving out the last line, doing the motions only. Repeat it a third time, leaving out the last two lines, doing the motions only. Continue in this manner until all lines are left out and you are doing the motions only.
- Vary the speed of presentation. Start at a normal speed. Repeat, going slightly faster each time. When it gets very fast, suddenly slow it down to prevent its becoming over-stimulating. Repeat three or four times, getting slower and slower with each repetition.
- Do the motions without words. Have the children guess which of the games you are playing.

TIME TO REST

It's time to rest, to rest your head	Put right forefinger in left palm.
Snuggled down in your own little bed.	Rock finger back and forth.
Covered up tight in blankets so warm,	Cover with left fingers.
Safe and cozy and away from all harm.	Bring hands to cheek, bend head against hands, close eyes.
(Rest a few moments.)	
In the morning the sun gives a peek,	Bring hands down; left forefinger (sun) straightens.
And says, "Ha, ha, you'd sleep all week,	Left forefinger waggles.
But now it's time to start a new day.	Left fingers uncurl.
Jump out of bed for school and for play."	Right finger out of palm.
First brush your teeth and wash your face,	Pantomime actions.
Fold your pajamas and put them in place,	Pantomime actions.
Get dressed and eat and then say adieu,	Pantomime actions.
Your teacher at school is waiting for you.	Finger hops up left arm.

(Continue in a hushed voice.)

Then at night when it's bedtime once more, Finger to lips; "Shhh."
And the lights are out and you've closed the door,
It's time once again to rest your head, Finger in left palm again.
Snuggled down in your own cozy little bed. Close left hand.

Optional (whispering): Now you can pretend you're that child
and curl up on the floor like you're cuddled in your own bed.

TEN LITTLE CHILDREN
(Tune: "Ten Little Indians")

One little, two little, three little children, Curl fingers into palms.
Four little, five little, six little children,
Seven little, eight little, nine little children,
Ten little children in bed.

One little, two little, three little children, Straighten fingers.
Four little, five little, six little children,
Seven little, eight little, nine little children,
Ten lift up their heads.

Music and Songs

Gentle and soft music is very helpful in promoting relaxation. As
the music quietly flows forth, children are enveloped in the accompanying rhythms and harmonies. Sometimes they listen quietly and reflectively, perhaps swaying their bodies gently in time
with the beat, achieving a state of repose and serenity. Other
times they can listen intently while they try to identify certain
sounds they have been asked to find. Still other times they can
listen while they lie quietly on mats or cots, with eyes closed,
letting the music lull them to sleep.

Meaningful Use of Recorded Music

Although children respond well to music, they respond even better to other human beings. Recordings, therefore, should not be
used as substitutes for adult facilitators or as easy escapes. In using
recordings, make sure that you are truly involved with the listen-

ing activity. Have on hand a few selections which you have listened to previously and which you have found to be especially
conducive to creating a restful atmosphere with a minimum of
emotional stimulation.

Use the following guidelines when choosing recorded music:

- For rest and relaxation, include some music without
  words. Trust in the power of the music itself to help achieve
  the desired atmosphere. You can help children to improve
  their listening skills by suggesting that they notice when
  the music goes to higher notes and when it goes to lower
  ones, when it gets louder and when it gets softer, when
  it plays slower and when it plays faster, and so forth.
- Avoid those recordings that have adult voices explaining
  the music.
- Select high-quality recordings performed by talented art-
  ists. Be discriminating.
- Avoid records with cute, artificially-pitched voices or
  voices that talk down to the listeners.
- Select recordings that have simple presentations. Complex
  symphonic musical arrangements may sometimes be emotionally overstimulating, especially to young children.
- Include some recordings that are made especially for children's resting and relaxation experiences.
- Avoid recordings with frequent changes of rhythm and
  pace.
- Familiar music is especially important, as it relieves the
  children from the repeated need to orient themselves emotionally to new pieces. Familiar music gives more immediate comfort and soothes restless children as well as
  adults. And since children always appreciate repetition,
  it isn't necessary to have a large collection of recordings,
  but rather a few carefully selected ones.

Improvising Songs

Even if you're not an accomplished singer, you can improvise
your own songs easily, making up words and singing them to

simple, familiar tunes. One advantage of improvising your own songs, in addition to being able to use those tunes that come most easily to you, is that the songs can be appropriate to the immediate interests and circumstances of the children for whom they are sung. You can come up with different words and ideas to fit whatever mood, activity, or learning you are trying to promote. And you can use words that fit with your own feelings, mood, and especially, your own personality. This kind of personalization makes your interaction with the children more meaningful to you and to them.

Sometimes it's good to sing lullabies after a story or other quiet activity. Sometimes you can sing lullabies for brief rest intervals during which children put their heads down on desk- or table-tops, or lie on rugs or resting mats. And sometimes you'll want to sing lullabies in the nap room while children are unwinding and getting ready for sleep.

GENTLY FLOWS THE PLAYTIME NOW
(Tune: "Twinkle, Twinkle, Little Star")

Gently flows the playtime now,
Gently flows the long, long day,
Time to rest your bodies now,
If you need help I'll show you how,
Close your eyes and gently try
To listen to my lullaby.

Gently flows the playtime now,
Gently flows the quiet time,
As you close your eyes so tight,
And pretend that it is night,
Sleep with one eye, sleep with two,
Sleep for me and sleep for you.

RESTING TIME
(Tune: "Frère Jacques")

Resting time now, resting time now,
    close your eyes, close your eyes,
Time for all the girls and boys,
To put away their games and toys,
Resting now . . . resting now.

Hear me whisper, how I love you,
loving you, loving you,
Time for all the girls and boys,
To put away their games and toys,
Loving you . . . loving you.

IT WAS TIME TO GO TO BED
(Tune: "Mary Had a Little Lamb"; very slow)

It was time to go to bed, go to bed, go to bed,
It was time to go to bed, and close my eyes so tight.
But I said, "Oh, teacher dear, oh, teacher dear, oh teacher dear,"
But I said, "Oh, teacher dear, it isn't even night."
And teacher said, "Just rest awhile, rest awhile, rest awhile,"
And teacher said, "Just rest awhile, lying down so still."
And so I said, "Oh teacher dear, oh teacher dear, oh teacher dear,"
And so I said, "Oh teacher dear, yes, indeed, I will."
I closed my eyes, and all was quiet, all was quiet, all was quiet,
I closed my eyes and all was quiet, and the world was quiet too.
And in the quiet I smiled a smile, smiled a smile, smiled a smile,
And in the quiet I smiled a smile, just like all of you.

Outdoor Resting Experiences

The various resting experiences that have been previously suggested can be conducted either indoors or out. The following suggestions are particularly appropriate for those times when the children are playing out-of-doors and you want them to gather together for a calming, resting experience.

Have children lie down on their backs, looking up toward the sky. Repeat the breathing exercises (page 92) four or five times. Then, ask everyone to close their eyes and listen to the outdoor sounds around them, being as still as possible.

✑ Clouds

If there are clouds in the sky, ask children to open their eyes and watch for shapes of people, animals, and other things that they can see in the clouds. Start the game by naming one or two shapes you observe. Give each child a turn to name a shape. After everyone has had a turn, suggest that everyone just watch how the clouds move.

When the children seem to be relaxed and composed, if you want to bring them back indoors you might suggest that they pretend they are clouds themselves. "A gentle breeze arises. The clouds get up and slowly, slowly, start floating toward the building. Clouds have no feet, so of course they can't be heard to make any sounds as they move."

Once inside, extend the restful episode by giving everyone a large sheet of colored construction paper and a piece of white chalk. With soft, slow music playing on the record player, suggest that the children draw some of the shapes they remember having seen in the clouds, keeping time to the music.

✑ Nature Search

Another relaxing and quieting outdoor activity is the nature search. Do this on a grassy area. Everyone searches in the grass until someone finds a live insect. Then everyone remains quiet and still while watching the insect.

After a few minutes, do some gentle movement activities in which children imitate the movements of the insects.

Besides insects, children can search for four-leaf clovers, pretty stones, dandelions, birds, or any number of other things.

✑ Watching Trees

On a cloudless day, instead of watching clouds, the children can watch trees:

1. Have the children lie down on their backs near any trees that may be in the play area.
2. Point out how the various branches and twigs move in many different directions.

3. Ask each child to pick out a limb or twig and try to hold one arm in the same position to the count of five. At the count of five, they may drop the arm and let it relax.
4. Repeat with the other arm, and then with each leg, one at a time.
5. Try extending all four limbs in directions similar to those of the tree. Count to five. Relax.
6. Repeat three or four times.

For silent resting, say, "Now the tree is going to rest awhile. Without moving, you may all rest awhile and be as quiet and as still as the tree."

This experience can be extended, as with the cloud watching, by drawing trees when returning to the classroom. An impressionistic variation of drawing trees involves the use of watercolors and soft, full brushes. As music plays softly, suggest to the children that they make the brush strokes go in different directions just like the limbs and branches of the trees they watched.

Creating a Restful Nap Time

Naps at school should involve security, regularity, and comfort for children. No matter what type of program is used during the rest of the day, no matter how open-ended the curriculum is, and how much freedom of choice the children are given, nap time should be arranged so that it is routinely the same each day.

The ideal situation would be to use a separate area for naps, where the cots are left up permanently. Each child's cot is left in the same place from day to day, the room has probably been planned for maximum restfulness, and there is not the distraction of seeing toys, games, and equipment that are reminders of other, more active classroom experiences.

If, as in so many nursery schools and day care centers, the cots must be stored each day until nap time, and then placed in a room that has been used for play and other activities, extra consideration needs to be given to the preparation of the room.

Basic considerations conducive to a restful environment have been detailed in Chapter Three, with suggestions for a dual-purpose room on page 40.

In setting up the cots each day, take care always to put them in the same places so that the children can have the security of knowing and learning to be comfortable in their own places. As many toys and pieces of play equipment as possible should be put away, removed from view, faced toward a wall, or taken out of the room if possible, to eliminate their distracting influence. This task can be made easier if the rooms used for napping are equipped with the minimum of furnishings to begin with. Since children thrive in rooms in which there is plenty of room to move around, sparse furnishings are no problem even during their play periods.

The After-Lunch Walk

So many times children are given their lunches and expected to engage in quiet activities (reading books, playing with puzzles, listening to music) prior to nap time. The problem is that food intake temporarily raises the blood sugar level and gives new energy to the body. Quiet activity doesn't use up this energy and when children are asked to nap some twenty or thirty minutes later, they are not yet ready to calm down. An after-lunch walk can use up that excess energy.

Following the noon meal, you can take children on a short, slow walk around the neighborhood. The walk should be paced just fast enough to use up that after-lunch energy, but slow enough and short enough so that they don't get fatigued. (On rainy days, you can take a walk inside the building.)

Make the walks interesting and something for the children to look forward to, by giving each a theme. For example, one day look for weeds growing through cracks in the sidewalk. Another day look only for brown roofs. Other days, find gray tree bark, brown tree bark, yellow-green foliage, dark green foliage, pebbles, house numbers, passing cars that are blue, passing cars that are tan, and so forth.

Establishing a Routine

Upon returning from the after-lunch walk, the children should use toilets and wash their hands. As they finish, they return by twos and threes to the nap area. You might have the children spend a few moments looking at picture books, listening to a story, or playing some quiet finger games before actually taking off their shoes and getting into their cots. Or you may want to help each child into a cot immediately upon entering the room.

Whatever routine you establish, it should be the same each day. After the children have been helped into their cots in a calm and soothing manner, it's important that you give some individual attention to each child—a little pat, a blanket tucked in, a smile—whatever is most natural for you.

No matter how well planned the napping is, there may be some children who are either too tense to relax or who rebel against having to nap in the first place. Some of this rebellion may stem from unhappy bedtime experiences at home. Some may come from the initial nap experience in school when being told to take a nap came as a surprise to those who thought school would be only a time for playing. Further, the strangeness of the surroundings and the presence of new people on the first day of school could have had a mildly traumatic effect so that all nap times are associated with that unpleasant first day.

Whatever the reasons for their rebellion, give children individual consideration, and work out a personal routine according to individual needs. *Routine* is the key word. There are many techniques that can be used to help children relax. Once you have found the one that works best for a particular child, use it to the advantage of you both.

Helping Children Relax

The following techniques may help children relax once they are already lying down on a cot:

- Place a small pillow under the child's head.

- Tuck in a blanket. Doing this means touching the child, and thus, reassurance.
- Stroke the child's back, shoulders, or arms gently for a few moments, and speak some reassuring words such as, "Just let yourself be still and quiet for a little while, and I'll be sitting in the rocking chair watching you," or "You may rest for just a little while, and then it will be time to play again." Sometimes being more explicit is helpful, saying something like, "After you nap, I'll help you put on your shoes and socks and then give you some juice."
- Say, "It's all right for you not to want to sleep. You must rest quietly while the other children are sleeping, but you don't have to sleep." Or say, "I know you don't want to sleep. That's all right not to want to. You can just rest instead of sleeping. But I can't let you disturb the other children, so try to rest very quietly."
- Sometimes you can help a child relax simply by having her or him change positions—perhaps face in another direction or lie on the back instead of the side. Try to learn in which position each child appears to be most comfortable.
- Walk from child to child and pat each one on the head. As you come to each child, say, "John is resting nicely," "Amanda is resting nicely," and so on.
- Anticipate! If you know there is a particular child who usually disturbs the others, have that child's cot close to the soundest sleepers or close to where you'll be sitting during the nap time.
- For an extremely restless child, a quiet place in another room, away from the nappers, may provide the proper environment to allow for relaxation, if not sleep.
- If you have tried many different methods, and if the child is physically well yet does not fall asleep, try to give that child some extra time each day for practicing relaxation techniques.
- If a child normally rests and naps with little difficulty, but appears to be restless on a particular day, check to make sure the child is not running a fever or showing some other indication of illness.

Wake-Up Time

The period immediately after awakening from naps should be just as much a routine as the period preceding and during the naps. When the environment has been properly prepared and the routines have been established with consideration for each individual child, most young children will nap from one-and-one-half to two hours. As they awaken, they should be helped to put on their shoes and socks and, if necessary, to go to the toilet. If the toilets are not adjacent to the classroom, an adult should accompany sleepy children to keep them from falling or otherwise hurting themselves. If no extra adult is available for these trips, children should go to the toilet in pairs, so that they can help one another. (If a teacher is generally alone during nap time, and the toilet is not adjacent to the room, a portable potty-chair should be available to accommodate those children who need to use the toilet while all of the others are still napping. Napping children, even if every one of them is sound asleep, should never be left alone.)

Only after all of the children have awakened and toileted and have their shoes and socks on should you turn on the lights and raise the shades. Some children need more time than others to wake up fully. Those who are more alert can help start folding sheets and blankets and stacking cots, while those who need more time can sit on a rug to stretch and move about at their own pace.

Children can snack after everybody is up, but it's a good idea to wait long enough to be sure they are fully alert. Sometimes it may be advisable to let the children play quietly with puzzles or look at picture books for five or ten minutes before serving a snack.

Whatever the routine, the fifteen to twenty minutes following nap time should be kept very low-key to allow for the varying rhythms of children and to give consideration to those who are slower in coming back to their normal pace and wakefulness.

Developing Inner Awareness

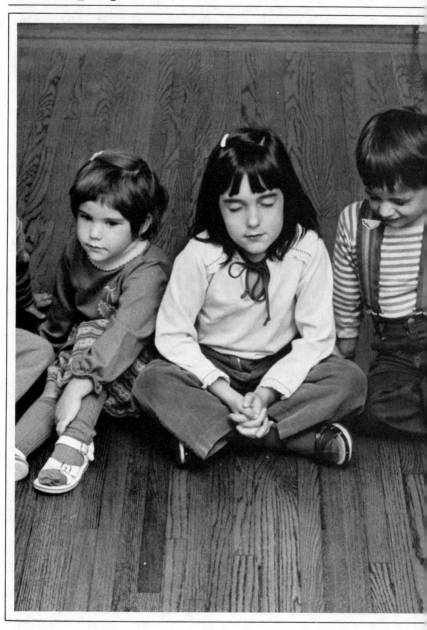

"Let's be very quiet and try to listen to sounds coming from outside the room."

I had gathered a small group of children around me and had asked each one to find a comfortable spot to sit down. I told them we were going to look for our own quiet, and that it might be easier to find it if our eyes were closed. After approximately one minute, I said:

"I closed the door and the windows. Now, let's listen only to the sounds coming from inside the room. (Pause.) Try to figure out what those sounds are. Don't tell me about them. Just think about them to yourself. (Pause.)

"Now (quietly) this is very hard. Put away all of the sounds that you heard from outside the room. (Pause.) Did you do that? (Pause.) Now put away all of the sounds that you hear inside the room. (Pause.) Have you put all those sounds away? (Pause.) Now, (in a hushed tone) close your eyes. Make yourself very loose and still. I'll count to three and then we can all listen to our own quiet. (Pause.) One. (Pause.) Two. (Pause.)

Three. (Pause.)

Wait two minutes, at least.

"Now I'm going to ask you to open your eyes very, very slowly. (Pause.) Look around at all your friends. Feel good inside of yourself. (Pause.)"

After this initial experience, I could intrude on a noisy, restless group and simply say, "Let's close our eyes and listen to our own quiet." Within two or three minutes the entire group would become relaxed and refreshed.

Heart Breathe—Techniques for Inner Awareness

Heart breathe is what I call simple meditative experiences for young children. The experiences involve being very quiet, listening to the inner self, and becoming aware of the heart beat and the breathing rhythm. Some heart breathe exercises are breathing experiences. Some are listening experiences. And some are a combination of controlled breathing and listening. All should be done with children seated. Aside from the tranquility to which the exercises themselves can lead, when children become aware of their own inner body functions they tend to develop a greater sensitivity to others. Experiences which help persons to become more sensitive to each other give hope to the possibility of a future in which there is deeper understanding, and thus less stress, between all living beings.

The Value of Breathing Exercises

By controlling our breathing we can control chemical balances in our blood that prepare the body for heightened or diminished activity. When we breathe in less—slower or shallower inhalations—there is a decrease in the supply of oxygen and an increase in carbon dioxide. Thus the activities of the nerves and the brain slow down, and the body is geared for rest and relaxation.

The exercises given here are planned for children from three to eight years of age. They are meant to bring about a moderate sense of relaxation and self-awareness and to maintain that level rather than to aim toward deeper, trancelike, meditative states. The operating principle is to begin with a short series of slow, deep breaths followed by a longer sequence of short, shallow breaths. You must take great care not to overdo these exercises with children. Too great an increase of carbon dioxide in the system will result in a reflexive action causing us to inhale deeply—even gasp for breath. This gasping for breath instantly changes the chemical balance in the blood as the oxygen in the blood increases, stimulating the nerves and brain.

◆§ Heart Breathe Number One

Have the children find comfortable places to sit and say:

> While I count to three, I want you to take a very deep
> breath and fill your entire body with air. Try to get the
> air into all the parts of your body. Then hold your breath
> until I count back to one again. While I count backward,
> I want you to let all of the air out slowly. After we do
> that three times, we'll do the same thing except that I'll
> count to two very quickly, and you will take very short
> breaths. Get ready now.
>
> One, two, three. Breathe the air into all parts of your
> body and hold it. Now, three, two, one. All the air is
> out.
>
> Again.
>
> One, two, three. Hold your breath now. (Pause) Now,
> three, two, one. All the air is out.
>
> Now we'll take little breaths.
>
> One, two.
>
> One, two.
>
> One, two. (Repeat six more times.)
>
> Now we'll take one more deep breath.
>
> One, two, three. Hold it. (Pause.) Now, three, two,
> one. All the air is again out of your body.
>
> Now we'll take little breaths again.
>
> One, two; two, one. (Repeat twelve times.)
>
> (Pause.)
>
> Now, just listen quietly to your own breathing, and just
> let yourself float around inside of yourself right there
> where you're sitting. Keep your eyes closed and listen to
> your own heart beat and your own breathing.

◆§ Heart Breathe Number Two

Do Heart Breathe Number One, and while the children are still
seated, say: "Now, just listen quietly to your own breathing while
I tell you a story. Keep your eyes gently closed. Let your eyes look

up even though they are closed. Look up instead of down. Is everyone doing it?"

Now, inside yourself, you're flying like a bird high up in the quiet blue sky. You find a soft, fluffy white cloud and let your whole self sink down into it. Just feel the soft white cloud all around you. It is fluffy and comfortable and feels just like a big pile of soft, fluffy cotton So soft. So quiet. So high. Slowly, you stretch out your wings. Wave them gently in the air. And then, through the cool blue sky, you fly back to me and open your eyes.

✑ A Heart Breathe Song

Usually, after a meditative experience such as the two preceding ones, I softly sing "Oh, Listening to My Love," which was inspired by the lovely song, "Listen, Listen, Listen, to My Heart Song," by Parmahansa Yogananda.

OH, LISTENING TO MY LOVE
(Tune: "Farmer in the Dell")

Oh, listening to my heart,
Oh, listening to my love.
Oh, listening to my heart song now,
Oh, listening to my love.

Our friendship always true,
Our friendship always true,
I won't forget, forsake, neglect,
I'll always be loving to you.

When you want to bring "Oh, Listening to My Love" to a close, sing each verse more quietly than the previous one until finally there are no sounds left.

Sometimes we make two small circles, the inner circle facing out and the outer circle facing in. The circles move slowly in opposite directions so that everyone has an opportunity to sing the song to everyone else. The movement is done very, very slowly.

Sometimes we sing the song holding hands in one big circle. Then I break the chain and start a serpentine twist until we are all wound together around one another. We finish the song in an expression of joy and closeness as we are all encircled. I vary this snake dance by asking children to go under each other's joined hands until they are in a big pretzel-type tangle and can no longer move. At this point, we usually fall to the floor feeling wonderful.

∞§ *Heart Breathe Number Three*

Say:

> You're just a little tiny baby on a smooth, soft, silky pillow in a little baby basket. You're so soft and gentle and quiet as you snuggle yourself down into the pillow. Your basket begins to rock slowly, slowly, first one way and then the other. Someone is singing a baby song.

ROCKING, ROCKING
(Tune: "Twinkle, Twinkle, Little Star")

Rocking, rocking, oh so slow,
Rocking, rocking, to and fro,
Little baby, soft and quiet,
Resting on your pillow white,
Rocking, rocking, oh so slow,
Rocking, rocking, to and fro.

Now, little babies, lie down on your backs and reach with your arms all about you, slowly stretching and reaching. Now reach with your legs all about you, stretching one leg out, then the other. Stretching them way, way out. Reach and stretch. Reach and stretch your arms now, then your legs. Reaching all about.

Now, lie very still and listen to yourself breathe. And if you listen very, very quietly, you might even hear the inside of you move. (Pause.)

Open your eyes slowly. Look around to remember where you are. Now slowly, slowly, sit up.

Sometimes, if the group has become too relaxed, I bring them back to a more normal state by a quick group sing or with two or three rounds of "Rock-a-bye Baby" with exaggerated dramatics.

✍ The Flower in the Meadow on the Mountain

This heart breathe activity is especially appropriate to use during springtime, or at any other time when planting activities and attention to growing things might be part of the curriculum. You tell the story and the children act the part of the flower.

You're a beautiful, graceful, purple flower living in the meadow on top of the mountain on the other side of the forest where the mocking birds live. Your petals are violet in the center, and all around the edges they are very deep, dark purple. Your petals stretch way out from your center, and the ends of each petal sway gently toward the ground. Gently. You feel the warmth of the sun shining on each one of your petals, and you look down and see the shadow they make on the ground. You nod your head just a little, and the shadow nods with you. You nod first one way and then the other, so slowly, so gently. And the shadow nods with you, too, so slowly and so gently. A bunny rabbit hops up to you and smells your petals. "Mmmmmmmmm," says the rabbit. "You smell so good." And then the bunny rabbit hops away. You watch and you watch and you see the rabbit get smaller and smaller, and pretty soon it's so far away and so small you can't even see it at all.

Now you stretch your long stem. It feels so good to stretch, and to stretch, and to stretch. And then to let go. You feel your roots as they stretch, too, deep under the ground. You wiggle them just a little, and then you notice that the sun is going down. Now it's going to get cold. Your roots, warm and comfortable under the ground, are all right. But your petals, out in the cold air with no cover on them, are getting very uncomfortable.

One by one you raise your petals up over your head until they all meet at the center. You hold them tightly together, close your eyes, and wait for another tomorrow.

The next morning, you awaken to hear the mocking birds singing. The sun is high in the sky. You wiggle your roots, you stretch your stem, and slowly and gently you unfold your petals to welcome the new day. All about you the mocking birds are dancing. You smile at them and say, "I know this is going to be a good day."

⋘ The Rock and the Stream

Have the children lie on the floor and close their eyes and, using a soothing, quiet, voice suggest that they get into their inside place where no one else can go. Pause after each sentence or two.

You are a rock in a quiet little stream. The water is flowing gently around you. You are heavy and hard and gray all over. Little birds come and sit on the part of you that sticks out above the water. Leaves and flowers that fall into the water bump into you, but you're so heavy, you don't move. The sun sparkles on the water like diamonds, and the sun's rays feel comfortable and warm on your back. But soon the sparkling diamonds disappear, and the water begins to look gray. The sky is now full of dark clouds, and you feel a gentle rain falling on your back. The rain falls harder and harder, and the stream is getting deeper and deeper and pushing up against you and all around you harder and harder. (Pause.)

Now you feel yourself moving very slowly and you begin to turn over. You roll down the stream, and the water is splashing all over you. You feel relieved when the storm is over. You roll to a stop, and all of the water on your back runs off. You look around to see your new home in the stream, and you like it just fine. The sun peeks out from the clouds, and once again you feel its warmth and shiny happiness.

Contributed by Janet Peters

Chapter Seven

Learning to Relax Muscles

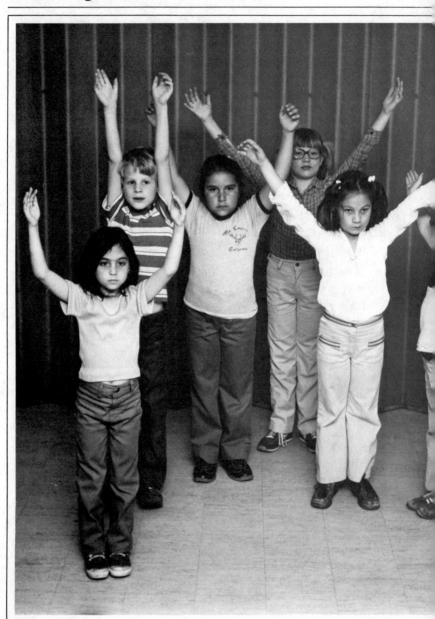

As the children gathered around me I said, "Today I want you to pretend that you are all new little baby trees waiting to be planted in the ground." I "planted" the children one by one, patted the floor around their "roots," poured a little imaginary water on the "ground," and said, "Oh, you poor little baby trees. You are so new and so weak you can hardly stand up straight. Listen, little trees, and I will help you to grow tall and strong. (Pause.) Feel your roots as they dig down into the ground. (Pause.) Feel the water coming in through the roots and making you stronger. Feel the sun shining down on your gentle limbs. (Pause.) Slowly, slowly, slowly stretch your limbs out to the sun. Feel them getting stronger and stronger. (Pause.) Feel your trunk getting taller and taller. (Pause) Feel your roots going deeper and deeper. (Pause.) I can see you are no longer weak, little baby trees. You have grown strong and tall and proud. You've become part of the earth below and part of the sky above. You give shade to those who are tired, food to those who are hungry, and wood to make homes for the homeless. Oh, trees. Oh, trees. You make the whole world a happy place."

As the children stood proudly and straight, basking in my approval, I suddenly said, "Ollie-kazoo. Magic. All of my trees suddenly turned into small, shiny flowers waving gently in the breeze."

Their instant release of muscular tension demonstrated the skills they had developed, over a period of weeks, of doing the types of exercises that are included in this chapter.

Relaxation as the Opposite of Tension

Many of the exercises and activities which are geared toward helping children learn the art of relaxation are closely tied to the principles of muscular control and release. The better we understand our abilities to control our bodies, the better we are able to use our muscles to relieve tension.

Isometrics and Yoga

Isometric and yoga-type (controlled postural positions) exercises can help children grasp the concept of relaxation as the opposite of tension. The exercises also provide children with a means of enhancing their skills in achieving total body control and relaxation. Such skills are beneficial to overall healthful development.

You can use the games that follow with children as young as three, but they can be effective for all children over three years of age. In using these exercises with three- or four-year-olds, you should limit the length of time and the number of exercises involved in keeping with their immaturity. Use discretion in determining how many you should use for any particular age group, since within each group the individuals can differ greatly. The key to planning should be to keep an activity slightly shorter and slightly simpler than you think might be appropriate. Gradually, as the group experience develops, you can lengthen the time involved and add to the number and complexity of the activities.

Individual Body Training for Relaxation

These exercises, which give the children experience in locating, tensing, holding the tension, then relaxing individual body parts, will help children come to understand they can control their muscles at will.

I find it best to do this activity with children sitting in chairs. The chairs can be grouped in a loose semicircle, a loose circle, or in a casual free arrangement. You might want children to remove their shoes for those exercises using feet and legs, though it is not essential that they do so.

When it is more convenient for a particular exercise, the children can stand. After some experience, they might try all of the exercises while standing. For a completely different experience, children can try doing the exercises while lying on the floor.

After each exercise, discuss with the children how they felt. Have them touch the parts that they were tensing. It will help the younger children if you touch the parts that are to be tensed beforehand. Touching those parts after each exercise provides instant feedback—reinforcing the kinesthetic awareness and memorization of the total experience.

RIGHT-HAND SQUEEZE

"Hold your left hand in your lap. Raise your right arm so that it is straight out in front of you, over your lap, with the palm of your right hand facing up toward the ceiling. When I count to three, make a tight fist wih the right hand. Hold it until I count back to one. One, two, three." All fists should be tightly clenched at this point. "Squeeze tightly. Three, two, one. Now you can let your hand relax and hang very loose." Repeat this two times.

LEFT-HAND SQUEEZE

Repeat the above exercise, using the opposite (left) arm and hand. Use "right" or "left" only for those children for whom the concept is easy. Three-year-olds and some four-year-olds usually do not have a good concept of laterality, and it's better simply to show them which hand to use each time.

TWO-HAND SQUEEZE

"This next exercise is very hard. We'll do both hands at once. Hold both arms straight out in front of you, palms up. One, two, three. Clench your fists tightly. (Pause.) Three, two, one. Now you can hold them open." Repeat two times.

ONE-ARM HUG

"Hold one hand in your lap. Raise the other arm and bring it across the front of your body so that your hand can grasp (take hold of) the other arm. When I count to three, squeeze your arm tightly with your hand. When I count back to one, hold on loosely. One, two, three. Squeeze tightly. Three, two, one. Loosely." Repeat two times; then do the exercise again reversing the position of the arms.

ONE-ARM TENSION
"Right where you held your arm, there are some muscles. This time I want you to make those muscles tight when I count. That means making them tense. Then when I count back to one, you can make them loose. That means making them relax. One, two, three. Hold. Three, two, one. Release." Repeat two more times; then do the exercise using the opposite arm.

TWO-ARM HUG
In the two-arm hug exercise, the arms are crossed over one another and both hands grasp their opposite arms at the same time. This is very difficult for three- and four-year-olds who have not developed a strong sense of laterality. Give directions as in One-Arm Hug, and do each exercise three times.

TOE-PRESS
"Press the ball of your right foot hard against the floor. One, two, three. Hold. Three, two, one. Release." Do three times with each foot. Repeat the exercise in a standing position. Children can discuss the difference in pressure between doing this exercise in the sitting position and doing it while standing. Whenever the opportunity arises, children can be made aware of the differences in the weight of their bodies depending on the position of their bodies.

BACK STRETCH
"Sit up very straight in your chairs. Rest your hands on your thighs. As I count to three, tighten your shoulders so that they almost touch each other, your chest sticks way out, and your back arches backward. One, two, three. Hold. Three, two, one. Release." Do three times.

STOMACH HOLD
"Sit up very straight in your chairs, hands resting on your thighs.

Draw in your stomachs very tight. One, two, three. Hold. Three, two, one. Release." Do three times.

SHOULDER SHRUG
"Bring your shoulders up toward the sides of your face. One, two, three. Hold. Three, two, one. Release." Do two times at the beginning; increase to three after children have done this exercise several times.

EYE WRINKLE
"Close your eyes tightly. One, two, three, four, five. Hold. Five, four, three, two, one. Release." Help children to practice making their faces taut for this exercise. Do three times.

MOUTH STRETCH
"Stretch your mouth as wide as possible, in a huge grin. One, two, three. Hold. Three, two, one. Release." Do two times.

LIP TIGHT
"Squeeze your lips together between your teeth as tight as you can. One, two, three. Hold. Three, two, one. Release." Do two times.

NECK STRETCH
"Sit very straight, with your head held high and tilted slightly toward the back with your chin sticking out, and stretch your neck tightly. One, two, three. Hold. Three, two one. Release." Do two times.

FINGER CLASP
"Fold your hands and squeeze them very tightly. One, two, three. Hold. Three, two, one. Release." Do three times.

PALM PRESS
"Hold your palms against each other and push very hard. One, two, three. Hold. Three, two, one. Release." Do three times.

FINGER PRESS
"Put your hands together so that just the fingertips and thumbtips touch. Press hard. One, two, three. Hold. Three, two, one. Release." Do three times.

WHOLE BODY HOLD

"Stand in front of your chairs, with your legs spread apart. Now make your whole body stiff. Feel the tension in the backs of your legs, in your arms, your stomachs, your backs, and your necks and faces. One, two, three, four, five. Hold. Five, four, three, two, one. Release." Do three times. After some experience with this exercise, children can gradually learn to do it with their feet closer together.

Total Body Relaxation through Tension and Release

After children have done the individual body part exercises a number of times, they can do this total body relaxation exercise.

To begin ask children to find comfortable positions on rugs, resting mats, carpets, or other spaces in which they have had previous resting experiences. They should lie on their backs and look up at the ceiling (or sky) for about two minutes, while everyone gets positioned. Say:

Wiggle your right leg. (Pause.) Now wiggle your left leg. (Pause.) Wiggle both legs. (Pause.) Now hold them very still. (Pause.) Wiggle your right arm. (Pause.) Wiggle your left arm. (Pause.) Now wiggle both arms, then hold them very still. (Pause.) Wiggle your shoulders up and down, then hold them still. (Pause.) Now wiggle your hips back and forth. (Pause.) Hold them still. (Pause.) Now wiggle all the parts of your body at one time very gently. (Pause.) Now hold them still. (Pause.) Now that you know where all the parts of your body are, I want you to listen to me, and have your body do what I say. I will have you make different parts very tight (tense) and then I will tell you to relax. When I say relax, then you make that part of the body very, very loose (release its tension) and let it be very still, quiet, and comfortable. I'll tell you each exercise just one time. Now you may all close your eyes, and I'll begin. You only have to listen to my voice and do what it tells you to do, just the way you did when sitting in the chairs.

Squeeze the top of your right arm with your left hand.
One, two, three, four, five. Relax.
Squeeze the top of your left arm with your right hand.
One, two, three, four, five. Relax.
Hug both arms at one time. One, two, three, four,
five. Relax. Put both arms straight along the sides of your
body.
Tense the muscles in your right arm. One, two, three.
Relax.
Tense the muscles in your left arm. One, two, three.
Relax.
Press your right toes against the top of the toes on your
left foot. One, two, three, four, five. Relax.
Press your left toes against the top of the toes on your
right foot. One, two, three, four, five. Relax.
Stretch your right leg out very straight in front of you
and lift it off the floor just a tiny bit while you tense the
muscles. One, two, three, four, five. Relax. Put your leg
down.
Stretch your left leg out very straight in front of you
and lift it off the floor just a little bit while you tense the
muscles. One, two, three, four, five. Relax. Put your leg
down.
Now you should begin to feel all loose and easy inside
of yourself. Your skin is beginning to get very loose on
top of your muscles. (Pause.) Everything inside of you is
beginning to get very, very relaxed and lazy. (Pause.) If
you keep on being very still and quiet, you might even
hear the inside of you move. (Pause.) Now I'm going to
tell you to tense and relax some other parts of your body.
Hold in your stomach very tightly. One, two, three,
four, five. Relax.
Hold in your seat (buttocks) very tightly. One, two,
three, four, five. Relax.
Push your chest up and hold your back very tightly.
One, two, three, four, five. Relax.
Squeeze your shoulders to the back toward the floor.
One, two, three, four, five. Relax.

Now squeeze your shoulders up toward the sides of your face and make them very tense. One, two, three, four, five. Relax.

Now just lie loosely and let all of the parts of the body that you have tensed and relaxed be very still and quiet. Think about how very loose the outside of you is by now. Think about the quiet of your own body.

Now squeeze your eyes shut tightly. One, two, three, four, five. Relax.

Squeeze your nose tightly. One, two, three, four, five. Relax.

Squeeze your lips very tightly. One, two, three, four, five. Relax.

Now. Make your whole head very tight. One, two, three, four, five. Relax.

Your whole body is very loose now inside of your skin. It's so loose that this next exercise is going to be very hard. I want you to think about filling up your whole skin with the inside of yourself. Take a very deep breath and tense your whole body. One, two, three, four, five. Relax.

Now just let yourself sink into the space around you. Your body is so light it feels like it's floating in the air. Your legs want to float up into the air. Your arms want to float up into the air. If you want to, you can let your hands float up into the air. Just keep your eyes closed and feel your life inside of you so relaxed. So lazy. So gentle. So relaxed. Breathe gently. Relax. Breathe. Relax. Take a deep breath. (Pause.) Now another.

Now let's go back to the beginning. Wiggle your legs gently. Wiggle your arms gently. Wiggle just your fingers and your toes. Wiggle your whole body. Sit up slowly; open your eyes. Stretch your arms up and around you. (Pause; allow time to stretch.) Now, when I count to three, you can stop being lazy. One, two, three. Everyone can be wide awake now.

At this point, allow time for various children to tell you how the experience made them feel.

Relaxation/Tension

One way to help children develop a solid understanding of relaxation as opposed to tension is to explore some of the words that are used to describe feelings of tension and the release of tension. You can use the words to lead children in whole body movements while sitting on the floor.

TENSE	RELAXED
tight	loose
stiff	limber
hard	soft
rigid	flexible
rough	gentle
tense	relaxed

Say:

Be the tightest person in the world. (Pause.) Now be the loosest person in the world. (Pause.)

Pretend the floor is the hardest thing you've ever sat on. (Pause.) Now pretend it's the softest thing you've ever sat on. So soft. (Pause.)

Rub the back of your hand as roughly as you can. (Pause.) Now rub it as gently as you can. (Pause.) (Continue in this fashion.)

✒ The Froggie

Here's a game that involves muscular tension and release.

DID YOU EVER SEE A FROGGIE?
(Tune: "Did You Ever See a Lassie?")

Did you ever see a froggie, a froggie, a froggie,   Children sit
　Did you ever see a froggie just sit in the sun?   on haunches.
Now jump my little froggie, oh froggie, oh froggie,   Children do
　Now jump my little froggie and let's have some fun.   frog jumps.
Now swim my little froggie, oh froggie, oh froggie,   Children do
　Now swim my little froggie, in the water so clear.   breast-stroke.

Now sit my little froggie, oh froggie, oh froggie,
Now sit my little froggie on your
  haunches right here.   Children sit on haunches.
Now sleep my little froggie, oh froggie, oh froggie,
  Now sleep my little froggie, right   Children lie down. Repeat several
  here in the sun.   times to extend "sleeping" time.
Wake up now little froggie, oh froggie, oh froggie,
  Wake up now little froggie, and let's have some fun.

Finish with first verse, or repeat entire sequence.

✍ The Fat Balloon

Say:

> I'm going to sing a song about a balloon. This is going
> to be a fat, red balloon that will float very high up into
> the air until someone sticks a pin in it. Then what will
> happen to it? (Pause for answers.) That's right. It will
> pop. What will happen to it after it pops? (Pause for
> answers.) That's right. It will probably just drop down on
> the ground and lie there all loose and empty. Now you
> can all pretend to be a balloon and blow yourself up.

THE FAT BALLOON
(Tune: "Go Tell Aunt Rhoady")

I'm a fat bal-loo-oo-oon,
A floating, soft bal-loo-oo-oon,
A rub-ber-y, round bal-loo-oo-oon,   Children puff themselves
Flying toward the top.   up and "float" lightly
                                        around the room.

I'm a big bal-loo-oo-oon,
A full of air bal-loo-oo-oon,
A floating, red bal-loo-oo-oon,   On the word POP!
Stick me and I'll . . . POP!   the children collapse
                                        onto the floor.

Little red bal-loo-oo-oon,
Out-of-air bal-loo-oo-oon,
Lying now so qui-et-ly,   (Repeat this verse for
Right where you did drop.   a longer rest time.)

Little red bal-loo-oo-oon,
Out-of-air bal-loo-oo-oon,
Blow yourself back up again   Children become
With all the air you've got.   balloons again.

Go back to the first verse and repeat the sequence.

✍ Grasshopper, Grasshopper

Say:

> Have you ever seen a grasshopper? Do you know how
> it jumps? Can someone show us how a grasshopper
> jumps? (Pause, while one or two children demonstrate.)
> That's right. It makes its legs very tight and then it lets
> go with a big jump, and it lands lightly on the ground.
> Then it tightens its legs again and starts all over. I'm
> going to sing a song while you can all pretend to be
> grasshoppers. The words tell you what to do.

Use a tambourine accompaniment, hitting a steady beat.
Have it get quieter and quieter until, when the grasshopper
sleeps, it can scarcely be heard. Then play it loudly again when
the grasshopper wakes up.   .

GRASSHOPPER, GRASSHOPPER
(Tune: "Pussy-Cat, Pussy-Cat, Where Have You Been?")

Grasshopper, grasshopper, hopping around,
Up in the air and back down on the ground,
Hopping so high and then sitting so still,
Hopping all the way to the top of the hill.

Grasshopper, grasshopper, I see you there,
Jumping and leaping way up in the air,
Then hopping to rest near the old wading pool,
Sleeping on green grass so tall and so cool.

Grasshopper, sleeping, your eyes closed so tight,
Sleeping all day and then sleeping all night,
Grasshopper, wake and start hopping around,
Up in the air and back down on the ground.

✍ Jiggling My Body

The first time you do this activity explain to the children that it is similar to doing exercises, except that you're going to make the exercises into a kind of dance. Demonstrate the different movements for them. Naturally, after the children have done this one or two times, all you will have to say is, "Let's jiggle our bodies," and start singing the song.

JIGGLING MY BODY
(Tune: "Oh Where, Oh Where, Has My Little Dog Gone?")

Jiggling your body to move all around,
Jiggling and shaking with me,
Shaking it hard to make it come loose,
Jiggling your body with me.

Twisting your head as you move it around,
Oh twisting and twisting with me,
Twisting it back, to the side and around,
Oh twisting your head now with me.

Stretching your arms as you reach for the sky,
Oh stretching and reaching with me,
Stretching way out and up high and around,
Stretching your arms out with me.

Lifting a knee and then kicking it out,
Kicking and kicking with me,
Kicking your leg to stretch way out in front,
Stretching it out there with me.

Other knee lifting and kicking it out,
Kicking and kicking with me,
Kicking your leg to stretch way out in front,
Stretching it out there with me.

Bending way down with right hand on left leg,
Bending and bending with me,
Bending way down to stretch near to the ground,
Bending way down there with me.

Bending way down with left hand on right leg,

Bending and bending with me,
Bending way down to stretch near to the ground,
Bending way down there with me.

Arms in the air and then touching the ground,
Touching and touching with me,
Touching the ground just as hard as you can,
Touching your hands down with me.

> (If children cannot touch the ground, change to
> "Arms in the air and then touching your legs.")

Standing on one foot with arms to the side,
Standing and standing with me,
Arms stretching far out to balance yourself,
Standing on one leg with me.

Swinging your arms from one side to the other
Twisting while swinging with me,
Twisting my head as my arms swing around,
Twisting your body with me.

Resting yourself as your arms hang down loose,
Resting and resting with me,
Arms hanging loose as you dangle about,
Resting your body with me.

Lying down now as you close both your eyes,
Closing your eyes now with me,
Let yourself loose as you lie on the ground,
Closing your two eyes with me.

> (Pause, then continue softly.)

Letting yourself just be loose on the ground,
Loosening and loosening with me,
Breathing your heat beat while loose on the ground,
Breathing your heart beat with me.

In addition to the above verses you can make up other verses that require students to hold particular positions to the end of the verse. Or you can have students hold positions by occasionally saying, "Freeze," while you pause for a few seconds.

ꠂ The Golden Feather

This story, which children act out, provides a gentle introduction to simplified, yoga-type exercises. The aim is to practice controlled postures which will enhance bodily flexibility, create understanding of how bodies work, and expand the ability to use bodies in healthful ways which can benefit overall well-being and help relieve tension. (See the Bibliography for books about yoga for children.) To begin, children can do the postural exercises in The Golden Feather while sitting on the floor. (You should lead students through the exercises by demonstrating the postures as the story goes along.) Later children can do the same exercises while standing. The Golden Feather works best when children become completely absorbed in the story, identifying with each of the characters.

This is a story about a feather. It was a very unusual feather because it was golden. It was a beautiful feather, just a little bit curved, and that made it look very gentle. I found the feather one windy day when I was walking in front of my house. There were leaves blowing around, scraps of paper, and weeds. And there was this feather. It blew right past my face, then tumbled around and went high up into the air, and then nose-dived right down on the sidewalk near my feet.

At first I didn't know it was a feather. I just saw this sparkling, shiny, golden thing flying around in the air. But when I bent down to pick it up, I saw that it was a feather, a real feather. It was so sparkly and shiny it looked as if it was made out of metal. But when I touched it, I could tell it was a real feather.

It was a very warm day, so, holding the feather in my hand, I walked over to a tree, sat down on the grass beside the tree, leaned back, and closed my eyes. I felt the feather in my hand, and touched it with the fingers of my other hand. It was smooth and gentle, smooth and gentle, and soon I felt as if I were the feather. (Pause.)

I'm a golden feather. I came from a faraway land. I've been carried by the wind all over the world. I've been

many places and seen many things. In the African
jungles I saw giraffes walking with their long necks
reaching toward the sky. Can you stand very still like a
giraffe with your long neck reaching toward the sky?

I said to the giraffe, "Oh, giraffe, giraffe. You are so
tall and wise. I'm just a lost golden feather. Can you tell
me where I belong?"

The giraffe, who did not ever make any sounds, just
shook its head on its long, long neck. No, the giraffe did
not know where I, the golden feather, belonged.

And then I went a little further and I saw big, giant
elephants walking through the fields. One very large
elephant saw me, stopped, raised its trunk way up high in
the air in a beautiful arc, and stood very still. Can you
pretend you are an elephant with your trunk raised high
in the air standing very still?

I said to the elephant, "Oh, elephant, elephant. You
are so big and wise. I'm just a lost golden feather. Can
you tell me where I belong?"

The elephant shook its trunk back and forth. No, it
did not know where I, the golden feather, belonged.

And so I went on to another place. On the edge of a
cliff I saw some beautiful, giant birds. They were bent
over, with their wings spread out behind them, getting
ready to fly away. When they saw me they stood very
still. Can you pretend you are one of those giant birds
standing bent over with your wings stretched out behind
you just getting ready to fly off into the air?

I said to the first bird, "Oh, bird, bird. You are so
beautiful and so wise. I'm just a lost golden feather. Can
you tell me where I belong?"

The bird continued to stand very still for a few
seconds. Then it said, in a very high, shrill, voice,
"Noooooooooooooo!"

So I went on to yet another place in another land.
Here I saw an ostrich, with a big, fluffy, feathery tail. I
said to the ostrich, "Oh, ostrich, ostrich. You have so
many fluffy feathers. I'm just a lost golden feather. You

are so big and so wise. Do you know where I belong?"

The ostrich lifted one foot in the air and just looked at me and didn't even answer. Can you be an ostrich with a big, fluffy, feathery tail standing on one leg just looking at me?

Then I said to the ostrich, "Please, ostrich. Please tell me where I belong." I guess it didn't know, because it bent over and buried its head in the sand. Can you bend over like the ostrich and pretend that your head is buried in the sand?

I decided to go to yet another land. There were many deer running down below. I went down to the deer, and they became very still. They were standing with their legs in a position as though they were going to run. But they held their heads up high and didn't move. Can you pretend you are one of those deer standing very still, but in position so that you can start running when you are ready to? I said, "Deer, deer. I am a lost golden feather. You are so graceful and wise. Can you tell me where I belong?" All the deer shook their heads slowly to tell me they did not know.

So on I went. I decided to try the fish in the ocean. When I came to the ocean, I saw a beautiful, rainbow-colored fish arching its back as it leaped over and under the waves. Can you pretend you're that rainbow-colored fish with your back arched just as you are getting ready to leap over the waves? When the fish saw me, I said, "Oh, fish, fish. You are so beautiful with all of your rainbow colors, and you are so wise. I am just a lost golden feather. Can you tell me where I belong?" But the fish didn't answer me so I went on to another place.

This time, along the seashore, I saw a very old giant crab. It had its arms and legs spread out in all directions. Can you pretend you are a giant crab with your arms and legs spread in all directions? When the crab saw me, it didn't move. I said, "Oh, crab, crab. You are so old and so wise. I am just a lost golden feather. Can you tell me where I belong?" The crab didn't even answer, and soon I decided that it didn't know where I belonged.

I went on to another land. I saw a long, slippery, slithery snake wiggling through the bushes. When the snake saw me, it stood very still. Can you pretend you're a snake holding very still? I said, "Oh, snake, snake. You are so slithery and wise. I am just a lost golden feather. Can you tell me where I belong?" The snake raised its head just a little and shook it back and forth, as if to say, "No."

So I went on further still. Then I came to this beautiful, very tall tree. Can you be a beautiful tall tree standing on the top of a hill? My, how tall and straight you look. I said, "Oh, tree, tree. You are so tall and so wise. Can you tell me where I belong? The tree swayed a big "No," and I was very sad.

I decided it was time to rest. I went down to the ground at the bottom of the tree. And there I found you. I'm so happy that I found you. You look so good and so wise. I am just a lost golden feather. Can you tell me where I belong?

Boys and girls, that is the story of the golden feather. I think it is asking if you know where it belongs. Would you like to keep that feather and tell it you will let it belong with you?

Pretend you are that golden feather. A child has told you that you now have a place to stay. The child even gave you a basket, with a bed of soft cotton in it, so you can rest when you want to.

Let me see by your faces how it feels to be a beautiful golden feather that isn't lost any more.

ᴥᔆ Extension of Golden Feather Exercises

The yoga-type exercises inspired by The Golden Feather can be done without the story. Once children learn about body control, they will begin to enjoy exercising simply for the feelings of accomplishment, relaxation, and tranquility. As their skills develop, children can do some of the following exercises.

In leading these exercises, you should demonstrate as you give the directions. Besides helping children understand what they are to do, your participation with them creates a real sense of group harmony.

1. Sit on floor, legs apart, bend head to floor. Hold. One, two, three. Relax.
2. Lie face down on the floor. Raise self with arms, keeping body straight. Hold. One, two, three. Relax.
3. Lie face down on the floor. Keeping legs together, raise them as high as possible. Hold. One, two, three. Relax.
4. Lie face down on the floor, body straight, arms extended. Keeping legs together and hands touching, raise both legs and arms. Hold. One, two. Relax.
5. Lie on back, body straight, arms at sides. Arch the back leaving a space between it and the floor, but not lifting the head off the floor. Hold. One, two, three. Relax.
6. Lie on back, knees bent, feet flat on floor. Slowly raise legs as far up and back toward head as possible. Keep legs together. Hold. One, two. Relax.
7. Same as above, raising back off of ground as feet are brought up. Hold. One, two. Relax.
8. Lie on back, body straight, arms at sides. Rise to sitting position without pushing with arms. Hold. One, two. Relax.
9. Sit with legs straight out in front of you, hands at sides. Keeping legs together and straight, raise them slightly from the ground. Hold. One, two. Relax.

Very young children respond best to these exercises when simple singing games are incorporated. Try the song that follows:

I SIT ON THE FLOOR
(Tune: "The Farmer in the Dell"; sung very slowly)

I sit down on the floor, and move my feet apart,
I bend my head down to the floor (pause),
Then sit back up again.
I lie down on the floor, and keep my body straight,
I raise myself with my two arms (pause),
Then lie back down again.

I lie down on the floor, and keep my body straight,
I raise my legs up in the air (pause),
Then put them down again.
I lie down on my back, and keep my body straight,
Raise legs and arms up in the air (pause),
Then put them down again.
I lie flat on the floor, and keep my body straight,
My head stays down, I arch (curve) my back (pause),
Then lie down flat again.
I lie flat on my back, and bend both of my knees,
I raise my legs up high and back (pause),
Then lie down flat again.
I lie flat on my back, and bend both of my knees,
Raise legs and back up very high (pause),
Then lie down flat again.
I lie flat on my back, my arms held at my side,
Without my arms I sit right up (pause),
And then lie flat again.
I sit down on the floor, my legs straight out in front,
I raise my legs a little ways (pause),
Then put them down again.

With a little practice, you can add exercises and make up your own rhymes.

◆§ Hang Loose

Sometimes when I want to get the children's attention and encourage immediate relaxation, I say, "Hang loose, everyone."

I immediately "hang loose" myself, and the children eagerly follow suit.

Because of the daily stresses we all face, hanging loose isn't as easy a task as it seems to be at first. Here's how I teach children to do it:

1. Stand comfortably with feet a few inches apart.
2. Now, forget about good posture, and let your head sink down into your shoulders, your shoulders sink down into your stomach, your stomach sink down into your hips,

your hips sink down into your legs, your legs sink down into your feet, and your feet sink down into the floor.
3. In this position, hang loose. Your arms are just dangling from your shoulders. If I push your shoulders, they'll move right back into position, sometimes moving to and fro a little until they stop. If I can do that to you, and if your body doesn't try to stop me, you are probably hanging loose. (The goal is to allow the body to "float," rather than to be held in a controlled position. I walk around the circle testing children to see how loose they are by moving their arms. If children are loose, a slight tap on the arms will make them swing to and fro, in a sort of bouncing movement.)

⋙ Rag Doll—A Hanging Loose Variation

The rag doll exercise is a traditional method of relaxing the muscles that even very young children like. The body is bent at the waist, and the arms and head are allowed to dangle freely. Repeat the exercise as many times as interest allows.

Say:

Let's all be rag dolls. Just let yourself hang loose, and I'll say the rag doll poem.

Ribbons and rags and cotton and thread,
They don't help me to hold up my head,
All I can do is bend over way down,
And be the funniest old rag doll in town.

My legs are so wobbly they bend at the knee,
I can't stand up straight as you surely can see,
My hands hang loose and just dangle around,
If I don't watch out I'll just fall to the ground.

Oh poor little rag dolls scattered about,
Oh poor little rag dolls all tired out,
Take a deep breath, very deep (pause), and let it out slow,
Now get up, try again. Come on, dolls. Let's go.

Once children in the group learn how to "hang loose" and be rag dolls, you can use this relaxation technique with them individually. If you spot a child who seems especially tense, you might walk up to him or her and suggest quietly, "Hang loose, Tina," or "Be a rag doll for a few minutes, Ronald," while the rest of the children in the class continue whatever they're doing. Done in this way, relaxation becomes a special little game, just between you and the child.

Chapter Eight

Expressing Feelings to Reduce Stress

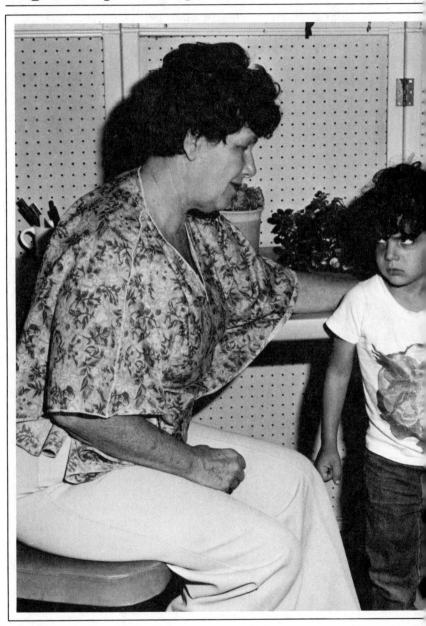

Gabe was very agitated. He had kicked another child— unusual behavior for Gabe, but it was the third time that week he'd been overly aggressive. The victim got much sympathetic attention from the two adult supervisors, and Gabe was totally ignored.

Soon he came into my office and told me he was very worried. I said, "That's O.K. Sometimes we worry about things." I went back to my work. Then he said he was unhappy. He kept trying to start a conversation with me (apparently to discuss his guilt), but I kept telling him that I was busy and that it was perfectly all right for him to keep being worried and unhappy. After about ten more minutes of ignoring him as I pursued my paperwork, I suggested that he could go to his classroom and be unhappy, since I was still busy. He left the room. Five minutes later he was back, and said, "I know. I know. I'm not unhappy. I'm first—, first—, first—. You know, that word you told me the other day." I said, "Frustrated." "That's right, that's right. I'm frus-

trated! Maybe I won't get so mad at people."

And Gabe was frustrated. He hadn't been pounced on for overreacting in anger. He hadn't been lectured or punished. He really was frustrated because his aggression did not get him the expected adult reaction. Gabe was an unusually intelligent boy, and he learned the lesson—he did not use that type of aggressive behavior against other children again. But he often told people that he was frustrated.

An Outlet for Feelings

If children are to realize quiet and serenity in their lives, they need a safe, nonjudgmental atmosphere in which to express the full range of their emotions. It's particularly important that children learn how to express and handle their negative feelings in appropriate, acceptable ways, rather than suppressing them.

Sometimes we may express our negative feelings in words or actions. At other times we may keep these feelings to ourselves, pretending they're not there. But when we suppress the expression of real feelings, we are being dishonest in our relationships with others, and we are possibly endangering our own well-being. Emotions involve certain bodily chemical changes, causing "butterflies" in the stomach, flushed faces, perspiring palms, rapid breathing, palpitations of the heart, and other symptoms. Less obvious are muscle contractions that accompany various emotions. If emotions remain unexpressed, those contractions, those tensions, continue far too long, creating a more or less constant state of stress which can have adverse effects on physical health.

Much of the tension experienced by young children is caused by the demand that they hold back their true feelings in order to please others. In their earliest years they hear such expressions as, "You don't really want that, do you?" or "You're too big to cry," or, "Don't you dare get mad at your nice little sister. She's only a baby," or "Don't be so impatient. That's not polite." These kinds of careless statements are all ways of saying to children, "Don't display your true emotions."

To help children become mature, emotionally secure adults, we should give them opportunities to learn to recognize their emotional reactions and help them to use their feelings constructively. Here is a four-step process I use when meeting with children's feelings:

STEP 1: RECOGNITION OF FEELINGS
One of the first steps in learning about handling feelings is to recognize them in the first place. Helping children to expand their "feeling" vocabulary is one way to help them recognize that

they are having a specific and identifiable emotional reaction to something. You can make such observations as: "I can see by the way your face looks that you are very angry." "I can tell by the way you are standing that you are very disappointed." "That must have made you feel very embarrassed." "You're really jealous of Tommy because he always gets the big trike first." Increase your own working vocabulary about feelings in order to help you recognize children's feelings and to express your own feelings to them. Spend several days observing children and jotting down the various feelings you see being expressed. Become aware of the various emotions you feel throughout a school day and add those to the list. Start out with a fairly small number and watch for times when you think that feeling is evident. Gradually add to your list. Children are capable of comprehending all of the feelings which adults experience. Feelings are universal. Children need help in recognizing and naming them.

STEP 2: ACCEPTANCE OF FEELINGS
Recognizing children's feelings must be followed by an expression of acceptance: "I can see by the way your face looks that you are very angry. That's O.K. It's all right to be angry." "I can tell by the way you are standing that you are very disappointed. It's all right for you to be disappointed. I get disappointed too sometimes." "That must have made you feel very embarrassed. I would be embarrassed, too, even though it was an accident." "You're really jealous of Tommy because he always gets the big trike first. Everyone gets jealous sometimes. It's really O.K. for you to want the trike even if you can't have it right now."

STEP 3: DEVELOPING HEALTHY CONTROL
Following the recognition and acceptance of children's varied feelings, you can begin helping them learn to develop control of their emotions.

To the child who was angry you could say, "I can't let you throw the vase," or "I can't let you kick me, but it's certainly all right for you to be angry at me because I wouldn't let you tear David's picture."

To the child who was disappointed, you might say, "I can't let you go home because that wouldn't be safe, but it's all right for you to feel sad because you're so disappointed. I get disappointed too sometimes."

To the child who was embarrassed, say something like, "I don't blame you for wanting to be by yourself for a little while. When you feel better, you can go be with the other children. If anyone says anything about what happened, just say it was an accident. I'll be there in case you need my help. They'll believe you, because everyone has accidents at one time or another."

To the jealous child, you can say, "Everyone feels jealous sometime. It's perfectly O.K. But I can't let you take the trike away from Tommy. You'll just have to wait your turn. I know you'll be impatient, and that's O.K. too. It's really all right to be impatient."

STEP 4: EXPRESSING YOUR OWN FEELINGS
Let children know that you have feelings, too. It's not enough to tell them that you sometimes have the same kinds of feelings they do. You need to express them out loud so the children can hear you. They can accept the feelings in themselves better, and thus bring them under control, when they can hear you say such things as: "Oh, I made a mistake. That really makes me feel frustrated. I'll have to do this paper over for the third time," or "I got a very sad letter today. It made me feel very unhappy, so I'm not in a very good mood. But I feel better telling you about it. I'm still going to be unhappy, but I think I'll forget about it while I'm helping you with the puppets," or "I'm sorry. I wasn't paying close attention. How embarrassing. After all, I'm supposed to be the teacher. I was thinking about a letter I have to write. I'll try to pay closer attention now. What did you ask me?" or "It makes me feel so excited to see everyone looking so happy and playing so nicely with each other. I want you all to know I love you very much."

Games about Feelings

You can use the two games which follow anytime as part of your music or creative movement programs. In playing these kinds of games, exaggerating the expressions and movements will be good examples to the children. After playing these games, you can ask questions such as:

>   What feeling is it easiest to act out?
>   Which feelings make you feel better when you play games about them?
>   Which are the hardest feelings to act?
>   What are some other ways we can let people know how we feel?

I like to end these kinds of games by having the children lie down on the floor, eyes closed, for a brief rest while they think about letting people know how they feel and about trying to find out how other people are feeling.

ᕦ *Show Me Feelings*

Have the children gather around you on the floor in a loose circle, semicircle, or other casual grouping. Tell them to get into comfortable positions. You might start the game by telling them to think of something quiet. Since they are accustomed to doing that, you would usually have their immediate attention and it sets the stage for this activity.

Say:

>   Show me on your faces how it feels to be happy. Don't tell me about it. Just show me on your faces. Show me on your faces how it feels to be sad. Show me on your faces how it feels to be disappointed. Show me on your faces how it feels to be jealous. Show me on your faces how it feels to be lonely. Show me on your faces how it feels to be surprised. Show me on your faces how it feels to be worried. Show me on your faces how it feels to be guilty. Show me on your faces how it feels to be excited. Show me on your faces how it feels to be afraid. Show me on your faces how it feels to be relaxed.

Add or substitute other feelings to meet the needs of specific individuals or the group as a whole. To vary this game, say, "Show me by the way you move how it feels to be happy," "Show me by the way you move how it feels to be sad," and so forth.

IF YOU'RE ANGRY
(Tune: "If You're Happy and You Know It")

If you're angry and you feel it stamp your feet,
If you're angry and you feel it stamp your feet,
If you're angry and you feel it,
Show us all how you would show it,
If you're angry and you feel it stamp your feet.

Other verses
If you're mean and you feel it scrunch your face
If you're silly and you feel it dance a jig
If you're scared and you feel it give a shriek
If you're sad and you feel it cry boo-hoo
If you're selfish and you feel it bow your head
If you're proud and you feel it stand up tall
If you're tired and you feel it give a yawn
If you're sleepy and you feel it blink your eyes
If you're loving and you feel it throw a kiss
If you're glad and you feel it smile a smile
If you're excited and you feel it give a jump
If you're relaxed and you feel it flop around

Children can be encouraged to make up their own verses.

WHEN I'M ANGRY
(Tune: "Here We Go Round the Mulberry Bush")

When I'm angry, I stamp my foot, stamp my foot, stamp my
foot,
When I'm angry, I stamp my foot, so early Monday
mornings.
When I'm sad, I cry some tears, cry some tears, cry some
tears,
When I'm sad I cry some tears, so early Tuesday mornings.

When I'm glad I smile and grin . . . Wednesday mornings.
When I'm afraid I cave all in . . . Thursday mornings.
When I'm confused I shake my head . . . Friday mornings.
When I can't decide I stroke my chin . . . Saturday mornings.
When I love I throw a kiss . . . Sunday mornings.

When embarrassed I hide my face . . . Monday mornings.
Disappointed, I pout my lips . . . Tuesday mornings.
When I hate I turn my back . . . Wednesday mornings.
When I forget I bow my head . . . Thursday mornings.
When I'm surprised I open my mouth . . . Friday mornings.
When I'm upset I bite my lips . . . Saturday mornings.
When I'm excited I jump around . . . Sunday mornings.

❧ The Blue Dress

The Blue Dress was written for the purpose of helping children
expand their emotional vocabularies and their understandings of
feelings. I've told the story repeatedly to the same group of children. They always respond with great empathy and look forward
with anticipation to the discussion period at the end. Such discussions provide ongoing clues to the child's growing awareness
of the impact of moods and emotions.

Rebecca was going to a birthday party. She was very
happy and excited because the party was for her friend,
Deborah. Deborah had moved to another house a few
weeks ago, and Rebecca was very lonesome for her. When
Deborah first moved, Rebecca pouted and frowned and
was very sad. When the invitation came, Rebecca was so
curious about who sent her a letter that she almost tore it
when she tried to open it in a hurry. Her heart gave a
little jump, and she was afraid that it was torn, but then
she was very relieved to see that it was all right after all.

Rebecca sent a note back to Deborah to tell her she
could come to the party. On the note she drew a picture
of two little girls with big tears coming from their eyes
because they were so lonely for each other. Rebecca's
mother said, "That's a good drawing. I'm very proud of
the way you draw." Rebecca felt proud, too, that her
mother thought it was a good drawing.

The party was in seven days. Rebecca was so impatient, she said, "I can hardly wait." Her mother said,
"You'll just have to be patient. But I have a surprise for

you. See this soft blue material? I'm going to make you a new party dress out of it." Rebecca said, "It is beautiful, Mother. It looks just like the sky."

The day of the party Rebecca got up very early and sang happy songs all morning. When she put on her new dress, it made her feel that she looked very pretty, and she felt good inside. She said, "Mother, I'll sit on the porch steps and wait for you to drive me to the party." She picked up the birthday gift she had for Deborah, carried it very carefully so she wouldn't mess up the big bow on the package, and went outdoors.

She started to sit down on the porch steps, but she saw something glittering on the ground by the rosebush. Curious, she ran over to the bush. She was disappointed to see that it was only a tiny scrap of shiny paper from a chewing gum wrapper. She bent over to pick it up and her dress caught on a thorn on the rosebush. When she moved to get it loose, she heard, "Tearrrrrr." Her stomach jumped inside of her. The dress had a big hole in it. She began to cry. Just then, her mother came out and said, "I'll be ready to take you soon." Then she saw what had happened. "I'm very angry. You shouldn't have been playing in that dress. I have no more of that material. I can't fix it. Come into the house. You'll have to put on something else to wear to the party."

Instead of going into the house, Rebecca sat down on the steps and began to cry. She was feeling very upset. Suddenly she heard a little bell going "tinkle, tinkle, tinkle." She looked up and there was a strange lady standing in front of her. She looked transparent, and Rebecca was frightened. "Don't be afraid, Rebecca," the lady said. "I'm your fairy godmother. Why are you crying?" Rebecca told her what had happened and said, "And my mother's mad at me, and I won't have a blue dress to wear to the party, and if I weren't so clumsy and careless I wouldn't have torn my dress, and I just feel terrible."

The fairy godmother said to her, "Don't feel so guilty,

Rebecca. It was just an accident. Now you wait right
here, and I'll be back in one minute." Right before
Rebecca's eyes, the fairy godmother disappeared. Rebecca
couldn't believe what was happening. She just stood there
with her mouth open in amazement. Before she could
even close her mouth, the fairy godmother was back.
And in her hand she had a piece of soft, silky, blue material that just matched Rebecca's dress.

"Where did you get that?"

"Oh, I just took a piece out of the sky. No one will
ever miss it." She placed the piece of sky on Rebecca's
dress and said, "Abracadabra blue," and the hole wasn't in
the dress any more. "Now don't you worry, Rebecca," she
said. "Just go tell your mother you're ready to go to the
party now."

Well, Rebecca's mother couldn't believe what she saw.
"Where did the hole go?" she asked. But Rebecca
couldn't tell her, because she didn't think her mother
would believe her, and she would be embarrassed. Her
mother felt very confused, but said, "Well, you can
explain it later. Let's go now so you won't be late for the
party." Rebecca was very contented as she sat back in the
car and relaxed. When she got to the party, she and her
friend Deborah were very happy to see each other again,
and they had a fine visit. They promised to see each
other again very soon.

That evening, when Rebecca was getting ready for bed,
her mother came into the room to help her. She picked
up Rebecca's dress and said, "Look here, Rebecca, what
did you do now?" There, right in the middle of the skirt
where the hole had been, was a big round black spot. It
looked just like a piece of night.

Rebecca said, "That's because the sun has gone down."
But her mother didn't understand.

You can ask the following questions to stimulate discussion:

Why was Rebecca lonely?
What kinds of feelings do we have when we're lonely?

Why did Rebecca and her mother feel proud?
How does it feel to be proud?
Why was Rebecca scared when she tried to open her in-
vitation?
How did that make her feel inside?
Why was she impatient?
How does it feel to be impatient?
What kind of surprise did Rebecca's mother have for her?
What kinds of feelings do we have when we're surprised?
Why did she carry the package so carefully?
How do you think she felt while she was carrying it?
What do you do when you are curious?
How does it make you feel?
Why was Rebecca disappointed?
How do you think she felt when her dress ripped?
Do you think her mother should have been angry?
Would you believe it if you saw a fairy godmother standing
in front of you?
How did Rebecca feel when she saw the fairy godmother?
How do you think she felt when she saw the piece of blue
sky?
Why was she embarrassed to tell her mother about the fairy
godmother?
Why was Rebecca feeling so contented on the way to the
party?
How did she feel while she was at the party?
How do you think Rebecca felt when her mother saw the
black spot on her beautiful blue dress?
How do you think Rebecca felt when she went to sleep that
night?
What would you feel like if you were Rebecca?

Any story can be made in a feelings exercise like The Blue
Dress, by simply inserting feeling words for each person and
action in the story. For example:

Once there were three bears. First there was Papa bear.
He was the biggest one of all. He felt *important*. The next
one was the Mama bear. She had just made the breakfast

porridge, and she felt very *satisfied* that it smelled so good. But she was a little *worried* because it was too hot to eat yet. The third one was Baby bear. Baby bear was very *impatient.* . . .

✵ Charades and Play-Acting

In Chapter Two, page 32, the game of charades was introduced. Children can play charades acting out feelings as well as stories. Groups take turns acting out emotions and guessing what emotions are being dramatized.

A closely related game is play-acting. You read a story and suggest to the children that with exaggerated facial expressions and movements, they can dramatize the emotions of various characters. As you read a story, the entire group can act out each part, or each person can do one sentence or one character. The following story was written especially for practice in expressing feelings. Other stories can be adapted for the same purpose.

One day I heard someone knock on my door. I was *curious* to know who was there so I opened the door. I was *surprised* that no one was there. Maybe I just imagined the knock on the door. I went back to the kitchen, and I heard another knock. I was *glad* that I hadn't been imagining things, and I went to the door again. I opened it very quickly, but I was very *disappointed* because again no one was there. I really felt *puzzled* and wondered if someone were playing a trick on me. This time I stayed near the door. Yes. I heard a knock again, and I opened the door very quickly. Now I began to get *worried* because again I didn't see anyone there. In fact, I began to feel *afraid,* and I was very *tense.* I sat right by the door and waited. And waited. I felt very *lonely* sitting there all by myself. And I was still *worried* and really *afraid.* Yes. There was that knock again. I was very *excited.* I opened the door immediately. And there, wagging its tail back and forth against the door was a little doggie. It saw me and got very *frightened* and ran behind the mulberry tree. I was very *relieved* that it was only a little doggie's tail that had been knocking on my door. I said, "Here, little doggie. Come here." And much to my *delight* the doggie came to me. I sat down on the front porch steps and patted the doggie's head. I felt very *happy* and *relaxed.* Then a lady came walking up to the house with a little boy. "Oh, there's our puppy dog," she said. The doggie ran to the little boy, the little boy picked it up, and they went away. I felt very *jealous* because the little boy had a puppy dog and I didn't have one. But I was also *relieved* that it wasn't a ghost that had knocked at my door. I went back into the house, closed the door, and went *happily* back to the kitchen where I had been fixing my lunch.

✒ Trust Walk

If children are to express their feelings openly in the classroom, they must be able to trust you and they must be able to trust each other, to feel safe from rejection or ridicule. The trust walk is a way to develop and demonstrate trust among children. Start with one pair of children at a time, so you can watch carefully as they learn the activity. As they gain experience in giving and receiving directions, you can have several pairs perform the activity at once.

One child wears a blindfold, another leads the blindfolded one around. The leader gives directions such as: "We're going through a doorway now," "We're turning left now" (or, "We're turning this way now"), "We're going to go up three steps," "We're coming to a chair," "We have an open space ahead of us. I'll tell you when we start coming to the wall," or similar comments that will help the blindfolded child walk with confidence.

Do the trust walk first in a very open, familiar area so that the blindfolded child knows in advance there won't be danger of bumping into anything. The blindfolded child and the leader can exchange places after a minute or so. Gradually the space can be more complex and the time can be extended.

When children have had much practice in this activity, they can try it outdoors. Outdoors, directions must include information about the ground surface. Be sure the blindfolded person is not led into areas where it would be easy to slip or stumble due to the terrain.

After everyone has participated, lead a discussion:

How did it feel to be blindfolded and not to see where you were going?

How did it feel to depend on someone else to show you where to go?

That feeling is called trust. What other times do we need to trust others?

What helped you most to know where you were going, your leader's hand or the leader's voice telling you where to go and how to step?

What would make it easier for you to walk with a blindfold on?

How do you think blind persons learn to move about by themselves?

Conclusion

It would be impossible to overemphasize the importance of the types of exercises included in this chapter. Suppression of true feelings can disturb physical and mental health and interfere with personal relationships. If we teach children, explicitly or implicitly, to hide and deny their real feelings, we are teaching ill health and anxiety. If, on the other hand, we provide children with ample opportunity to express their feelings, even the most negative ones, we are aiding their full, wholesome development as human beings.

Bibliography

Chapter One: Think of Something Quiet

Albrecht, Karl. *Stress and the Manager: Making It Work for You.* Englewood Cliffs, N.J.: Prentice-Hall, 1979.

Ayres, Jean A. *Sensory Integration and Learning Disorders.* Los Angeles: Western Psychological Services, 1972.

Bergan, John R., and Henderson, R.W. *Child Development.* Columbus, Ohio: Charles E. Merrill, 1979.

Brown, K., and Cooper, S. J., eds. *Chemical Influences on Behavior.* New York: Academic Press, 1979.

Capon, Jack. *Perceptual Motor Development: Balance Activities.* Belmont, Calif.: Pitman Learning, 1974.

Cherry, Clare. *Creative Movement for the Developing Child.* Rev. ed. Belmont, Calif.: Pitman Learning, 1971.

_____ , Harkness, B., and Kuzma, K. *Nursery School and Day Care Management Guide.* Rev. ed. Belmont, Calif.: Pitman Learning, 1979.

Corballis, C. and Beale, I. L. *The Psychology of Left and Right.* New York: Halsted Press, 1946.

Depue, Richard A., ed. *The Psychobiology of the Depressive Disorders: Implications for the Effect of Stress.* New York: Academic Press, 1979.

Feingold, Ben. *Why Your Child Is Hyperactive.* New York: Random House, 1975.

Feldenkrais, Morris. *Body and Mature Behavior.* New York: International Universities Press, 1970.

Freeman, L.; Sugarman, Daniel A. *The Search for Serenity.* New York: Macmillan, 1970.

Gil, David G. *Violence Against Children.* Cambridge, Mass.: Harvard University Press, 1970.

Insel, Paul M., and Lindgren, H. C. *Too Close for Comfort: The Psychology of Crowding.* Englewood Cliffs, N.J.: Prentice-Hall, 1978.

Jourard, Sidney M. "An Exploratory Study of Body Accessibility." *British Journal of Social and Clinical Psychology* 5 (1966): 221–31.

Jung, Carl G. *Modern Man in Search of a Soul.* New York: Harcourt, Brace Jovanovich, 1955.

Knapp, Mark L. *Nonverbal Communication in Human Interaction.* New York: Holt, Rinehart and Winston, 1972.

Levine, Sol, and Scotch, Norman A. *Social Stress.* Chicago: Aldine, 1970.

Luce, Gay Gaer. *Body Time: Physiological Rhythms and Social Stress.* New York: Pantheon Books, 1971.

McGough, Elizabeth. *Your Silent Language.* New York: Morrow, 1974.

Mehrabian, Albert. *Silent Messages.* Belmont, Calif.: Wadsworth, 1971.

Montagu, Ashley. *Touching: The Human Significance of the Skin.* New York: Columbia University Press, 1971.

Nagi, Saad Z. *Child Maltreatment in the United States.* New York: Columbia University Press, 1977.

Rogers, Carl. *On Becoming a Person.* Boston: Houghton Mifflin, 1961.

Selye, H. *Stress Without Distress.* Philadelphia: J. B. Lippincott, 1974.

————. *Stress of Life.* New York: McGraw-Hill, 1956.

Sheppard, G. Kellam; Branch, J. D.; Khazan, C. A.; and Ensminger, M. E. *Mental Health and Going to School.* Chicago: University of Chicago Press, 1975.

Singer, Jerome. "Fantasy: The Foundation of Serenity." *Psychology Today* 10 (1976): 32–37.

Smith, Lendon, M.D. *Feed Your Kids Right.* New York: McGraw-Hill, 1979.

————. *Improving Your Child's Behavior Chemistry.* Englewood Cliffs, N.J.: Prentice-Hall, 1976.

Szasz, Suzanne. *The Body Language of Children.* New York: W. W. Norton, 1978.

Valett, Robert. *Remediation of Learning Disabilities.* Belmont, Calif.: Pitman Learning, 1974.

Walker, C. Eugene. *Learn to Relax.* Englewood Cliffs, N.J.: Prentice-Hall, 1975.

Westman, Jack C. *Child Advocacy: New Professional Roles for Helping Families.* New York: Free Press, 1979.

White, Burton L. *The First Three Years of Life.* Englewood Cliffs, N.J.: Prentice-Hall, 1975.

Wittrock, Merl. *The Human Brain.* Englewood Cliffs, N.J.: Prentice-Hall, 1977.

Wunderlich, Ray C., M.D. *Kids, Brains, and Learning.* St. Petersburg, Fla.: Johnny Reads, 1970.

Chapter Two: Communicating with Children

Fromm, Erich. *The Art of Loving.* New York: Harper & Row, 1956.

Gibb, Jack R. *Trust: A New View of Personal and Organizational Development.* Los Angeles: Guild of Tutors Press, 1978.

Moustakas, Clark E. *Finding Yourself, Finding Others.* Englewood Cliffs, N.J.: Prentice-Hall, 1975.

Scott, Louise Binder. *Learning Time with Language Experiences for Young Children.* New York: McGraw-Hill, 1968.

Chapter Three: Creating Wholesome Environments

Cherry, Clare. *Creative Play for the Developing Child.* Belmont, Calif.: Pitman Learning, 1976.

————. *Creative Art for the Developing Child.* Belmont, Calif.: Pitman Learning, 1972.

_____. *Nursery School Bulletin Boards*. Belmont, Calif.: Pitman Learning, 1974.

Chapter Four: Responding to Stress

For Children
If parents are getting (or have gotten) a divorce:
Hazen, Barbara Shook. *Two Homes to Live In: A Child's-Eye View of Divorce*. New York: Human Sciences Press, 1978.
Lexau, Joan. *Emily and the Klunky Baby and the Next-Door Dog*. New York: Dial Press, 1972.
Mann, Peggy. *My Dad Lives in a Downtown Hotel*. Garden City, N.Y.: Doubleday, 1973.
Perry, Patricia,, and Lynch, Marietta. *Mommy and Daddy Are Divorced*. New York: Dial Press, 1978.
Rogers, Helen Spelman. *Morris and His Brave Lion*. New York: McGraw-Hill, 1975.
Simon, Norma. *All Kinds of Families*. Chicago: Albert Whitman, 1976.
Zolotow, Charlotte. *A Father Like That*. New York: Harper & Row, 1971.

About a parent's remarriage:

Clifton, Lucille. *Everett Anderson's 1-2-3*. New York: Holt, Rinehart and Winston, 1977.

When children are ill/hospitalized:

Bemelmans, Ludwig. *Madeline*. New York: Penguin, 1977.
Lexau, Joan. *Benjie On His Own*. New York: Dial Press, 1970.
McPhail, David. *The Bear's Toothache*. Boston: Little, Brown, 1972.
Rey, Margret, and Rey, H. A. *Curious George Goes to the Hospital*. Boston: Houghton Mifflin, 1966.
Sharmat, Marjorie Weinman. *I Want Mama*. New York: Harper & Row, 1974.
Silverstein, Alvin, and Silverstein, Virginia B. *Itch, Sniffle and Sneeze: All About Asthma, Hay Fever, and Other Allergies*. New York: Four Winds Press, 1978.
Weber, Alfons. *Elizabeth Gets Well*. New York: Thomas Y. Crowell, 1970.
Wiseman, Bernard. *Morris Has a Cold*. New York: Dodd Mead, 1978.

A new baby in the home:

Arnstein, Helene S. *Billy and Our New Baby*. New York: Human Sciences Press, 1973.
Greenfield, Eloise. *She Come Bringing Me That Little Baby Girl*. Philadelphia: J.B. Lippincott, 1974.
Jordan, June. *New Life: New Room*. New York: Thomas Y. Crowell, 1975.
Wolde, Gunilla. *Betsy's Baby Brother*. New York: Random House, 1975.

Dealing with death:

Bernstein, Joanne E., and Gullo, Stephen V. *When People Die*. New York: E. P. Dutton, 1977.
Fassler, Joan. *My Grandpa Died Today*. New York: Human Sciences Press, 1971.
Miles, Miska. *Annie and the Old One*. Boston: Little, Brown, 1971.
Stein, Sara Bonnett. *About Dying*. New York: Walker, 1974.

When animals or pets die:

Carrick, Carol. *The Foundling*. New York: Seabury Press, 1977.
Tobias, Tobi. *Petey*. New York: G. P. Putnam's Sons, 1978.
Viorst, Judith. *The Tenth Good Thing About Barney*. New York: Atheneum, 1971.

Fears, frustrations, anger, and general concerns:

Blaine, Marge. *The Terrible Thing That Happened at Our House*. New York: Parents' Magazine Press, 1975.
Breinburg, Petronella. *Shawn Goes to School*. New York: Thomas Y. Crowell, 1974.
Fassler, Joan. *The Boy with a Problem*. New York: Human Sciences Press, 1971.
————. *Don't Worry Dear*. New York: Human Sciences Press, 1971.
Grollman, Sharon H. *More Time to Grow: Explaining Mental Retardation to Children: A Story*. Boston: Beacon Press, 1977.
Kantrowitz, Mildred. *Maxie*. New York: Parents' Magazine Press, 1970.
Preston, Edna M. *The Temper Tantrum Book*. New York: Viking Press, 1969.
Sendak, Maurice. *Where the Wild Things Are*. New York: Harper & Row, 1963.
Showers, Paul. *A Book of Scary Things*. Garden City, N.Y.: Doubleday, 1977.
Simon, Norma. *I Was So Mad!* Chicago: Albert Whitman, 1974.
Viorst, Judith. *Alexander and the Terrible, Horrible, No Good, Very Bad Day*. New York: Atheneum, 1976.

Weather disasters and fire:

Anderson, Lonzo. *The Day the Hurricane Happened*. New York: Charles Scribner's Sons, 1974.
Ets, Marie Hall. *Gilberto and the Wind*. New York: Viking Press, 1963.
Gramatky, Hardie. *Little Toot on the Mississippi*. New York: G. P. Putnam's Sons, 1973.
Schick, Eleanor. *City in the Winter*. New York: Macmillan, 1973.
Zolotow, Charlotte. *The Storm Book*. New York: Harper & Row, 1952.

For Adults

Arnstein, Helen S. *What to Tell Your Child about Birth, Illness, Death, Divorce and Other Family Crises*. New York: Condor Publishing, 1978.
Dunn, Judy. *Distress and Comfort*. Cambridge, Mass.: Harvard University Press, 1977.

Fassler, Joan. *Helping Children Cope: Mastering Stress through Books and Stories.* New York: Free Press, 1978.

Grollman, E. A. *Explaining Death to Children.* Boston: Beacon Press, 1969.

Wolman, Benjamin B. *Children's Fears.* New York: Grosset & Dunlap, 1978.

Chapter Five: Getting the Most from Rest Time

Cartwright, Rosalind D. *A Primer on Sleep and Dreaming.* Reading, Mass.: Addison-Wesley, 1978.

Cromwell, Liz and Hibner, Dixie. *Finger Frolics: Fingerplays for Young Children.* Highland Park, N.J.: Gryphon House, 1976.

Deming, Richard. *Sleep, Our Unknown Life.* New York: Elsevier-Nelson, 1972.

Doan, Eleanor. *Fascinating Finger Fun.* Grand Rapids, MI.: Zondervan, 1972.

Hall, Adelaide. *Finger Plays: An Activity Book of Games, Rhymes, and Pantomimes.* New York: Golden Press, 1964.

Hogstrom, Daphne. *Little Boy Bue: Fingerplays Old and New.* New York: Golden Press, 1976.

Kelly, Charles P. *The Natural Way to Healthful Sleep.* New York: Grammarcy (by arrangement with Crown Publishers), 1961.

Record:

Hallum, Rosemary. *Finger Play Fun.* Baldwin, N.Y.: Educational Activities, 1979.

Chapter Six: Developing Inner Awareness

Benson, Herbert. *The Relaxation Response.* New York: Morrow, 1975.

Bloomfield, Harold H.; Cain, M. P.; Jaffe, D. T.; and Kory, R. B. *T.M.: Discovering Inner Energy and Overcoming Stress.* New York: Delacorte Press, 1975.

LeShan, Lawrence. *How to Meditate: A Guide to Self-Discovery.* Boston: Little, Brown, 1974.

Ornstein, Robert E. *The Psychology of Consciousness.* 2d. ed. New York: Harcourt Brace Jovanovich, 1977.

Samples, Bob. *The Metaphoric Mind: A Celebration of Creative Consciousness.* Reading, Mass.: Addison-Wesley, 1976.

Tulku, Tarthang. *Gesture of Balance: A Guide to Awareness, Self-Healing, and Meditation.* Emeryville, Calif.: Dharma, 1976.

Yogananda, Paramahansa. *Cosmic Chants: Words and Music of Sixty Spiritualized Songs.* 6th ed. Los Angeles: Self-Realization Fellowship, 1974.

Chapter Seven: Learning to Relax Muscles

Barr, Beverly. *Exercise Games for Children and Parents.* New York: Drake, 1978.

Capon, Jack. *Perceptual Motor Development: Balance Activities.* Belmont, Calif.: Pitman Learning, 1975.

Carr, Rachel. *Be a Frog, a Bird, or a Tree.* New York: Harper & Row, 1972.

Da Liu. *Taoist Health Exercise Book.* New York: Links Books, 1974.

Davis, Maetta. "Isometric Conditioning Exercise." *Academic Therapy* XI, Fall 1975, pp. 65–70.

Frostig, M. *Movement Education.* Chicago: Follet, 1970.

Hendricks, C.G., and Wills, Russell. *The Centering Book: Awareness Activities for Children, Parents, and Teachers.* Englewood Cliffs, N.J.: Prentice-Hall, 1975.

Hopkins, Laura J., and Thomas. "Yoga in Psychomotor Training." *Academic Therapy* XI, Summer 1976, pp. 461–465.

Kephart, Newell C. *The Slow Learner in the Classroom.* Columbus, Ohio: Charles E. Merrill, 1971.

Maisel, Edward. *Tai Chi for Health.* New York: Holt, Rinehart and Winston, 1972.

Marshall, Lyn. *Yoga for Your Children.* New York: Schocken Books, 1979.

Ross, Karen. *The New Manual of Yoga.* New York: Arco, 1977.

Torbert, Marianne. *Follow Me: A Handbook of Movement Activities for Children.* Englewood Cliffs, N.J.: Prentice-Hall, 1980.

Chapter Eight: Expressing Feelings to Reduce Stress

Brown, George Isaac. *Human Teaching for Human Learning.* New York: Viking Press, 1971.

Castillo, Gloria A. *Left-Handed Teaching: Lessons in Affective Education.* 2d ed. New York: Holt, Rinehart and Winston, 1978.

Dunn, Judy. *Feelings.* Mankato, Minn.: Creative Education, 1970.

Gaylin, Willard. *Feelings: Our Vital Signs.* New York: Harper & Row, 1979.

Hendricks, C. Gaylord, and Fadiman, James, eds. *Transpersonal Education.* Englewood Cliffs, N.J.: Prentice-Hall, 1976.

Jenson, Larry C., and Wells, M. Gawain. *Feelings: Helping Children Understand Emotions.* Salt Lake City: Brigham University Press, 1979.

Krishnamurti, Jiddu. *Education and the Significance of Life.* New York: Harper & Row, 1953.

Wood, John T. *How Do You Feel? A Guide to Your Emotions.* Englewood Cliffs, N.J.: Prentice-Hall, 1974.

Index

A

Abuse, *see* Child Abuse
Achievement (standards for), 61
Activities
    alternating rhythms of, 72
    motor, *see* Exercises; Movement
    outdoor, 83–85, 86
    physical, 10
    quieting, 6
    recognition of need for, 10
    relaxing, 10, 84
    sedentary, 51
    vigorous, 51
Acoustics, 36
Additive-free diet, 13
Adult facilitator, 72
AFTER-LUNCH WALK, 86
Air control, 36, 38
Alcoholism, 3
Alone box, 41
Alone place, 41
American Humane Association, 3
ANGELS IN THE SNOW, 54–55
AND EVERYONE WAS SOUND
    ASLEEP, 75–77
Anticipatory interference, 50
Anxiety, *see* Stress
Archetypal needs, 7
Arm movements, *see also* Muscular
    exercises
    as relaxant, 78
Arrangements
    central room plan, 39, 40
    loose, 53
    physical, 52–53
Atmosphere (calm, relaxed), 1, 4
    see also Environment
Auditory discrimination, 8

Awareness
    Golden rule of, 6
    inner, 4, 5, 12
    self, *see* Self-awareness

B

BABY, BABY IN YOUR BED, 78
Balance, 14
BARREL BOX, 41–42
THE BEAR WENT OVER BANANA,
    57–58
Bedtime, 87
Behavior
    disruptive, 13
    hyperactive, 12, 13, 40, 51
    stress-related, 10
    tense, 13
BEHIND-THE-FURNITURE-PLACES,
    42
Benches, 43
Bending, 9
Bilateral movements, *see* Laterality
Biochemical uniqueness, 12
Block places, 43
Blood
    chemical balance in, 92
    circulation, 73
Blood sugar, 10, 12–13
THE BLUE DRESS, 127–130
Body
    control of, 11, 14, 112, 115
    exercises for, 99–119
    locating parts of, 100
    relaxing parts of, 100–104
    rhythms of, 10
    training of, 100–104
Body language, *see* Communication,
    nonverbal

Brain hemispheres, 11
Breathing, *see also* Heart Breathe
    and chemical balance, 92
    controlled, 92
    exercises, 8, 92
    rapid, 122
    and relaxation, 55
    and resting, 73
    and self-awareness, 92
    rhythm of, 92
Bulletin boards, 37
Busing, 2

C

Cadmium poisoning, 13
Camaraderie, 49
Carbon dioxide, 92
Caring relationships, 6, 7
Central room arrangement plan, 39,
    40
Chairs, 43–44
CHARADES, 32
Chemicals, 13
    balance of, 92
    and emotions, 122
Circles (groups of children in), 42
Child advocacy, 3
Child abuse, 3, 63
Children
    abuse of, 3, 63
    control of, 3
    depressed, 3, 45
    development of, 8–15
    differences in, 10
    and fears, 61, 63, 65, 67
    passive, 63
    planning for groups of, 10
    out-of-control, 13, 58–59
    protection of, 3
    school age, 4
    stress in, 2–5
    very young, 118
Classes (methodology), 4
CLAY PLACES, 45

Clay (therapeutic effect of), 45
CLOTH CORNERS, 42
Color (in environment), 36
Communication
    awareness of, 20
    checklist for, 20–22
    effective, 19
    encouragement of, 21
    facial expressions, 22
    instant feedback of, 20
    games for, 24–33
    gestures, 22
    guidelines for, 20–22
    importance of, 20
    interpretation of, 22
    natural, 39
    nonverbal, 29–33
    with parents, 61–62
    relevance of, 21
    simplicity of, 21
    things to avoid, 22
    and touching, 22, 23–26
    and trust, 21–23
Conversations
    natural, 39
    nonverbal, 31
Cots, 40–41, 85–86, 87–88, 89
Crawling, 9, 14, 15
Creative movement, *see* Movement
Cross-laterality, *see* Laterality
Cultural differences, 3
Curriculum, 6

D

Death, 60
Depression, 3, 45
Despair, 2
Development
    balanced, 10
    handicaps of, 3
    imbalanced, 10
    natural, 10
    progress of, 8
    retarded, 10

Development *cont'd*
  wholesome, 133
DID YOU EVER SEE A FROGGIE,
  107–108
Diet (additive-free), 13
Disabilities
  learning, 10
  physical, 3
Discipline, 4
Divorce, 2
Dominance, *see* Laterality
Drawing corner, 44–45
Drawing table, 44
Drug addiction, 3
Dual-purpose room, 40–41

E

Economic pressure, 2
Ego strength, 11
Emergency procedures for out-of-
  control behavior, 58–59
Emotional tension (causes of), 51
Emotions, *see also* Feelings
  and chemical changes, 122
  and fatigue, 52, 53
  loss of control, 49
  recognition of, 122
  signs of, 122
  tenor of, 51
  and vigorous physical exercise,
    51
Environment, 35–47
  abusive, 63
  acoustics, 36
  alone places, 41–46
  bulletin boards, 37, 39
  calming effect of central room
    arrangement plan, 39, 40
  changing of, 4
  colors, 36, 42
  conducive to sleep, 40
  deprived, 63
  dual-purpose room, 40–41
  factors to be considered, 8

Environment *cont'd*
  flexibility, 39–40
  glare, 36
  humidity, 36, 37
  imagination space, 37
  learning, 37
  lighting, 36
  noise, 36
  planning involvement in, 40
  physical, 5
  polluted, 13
  psychological, 5
  relaxing, 16–17, 38
  room arrangements, 38–39
  and serenity, 36–37
  and sense of security, 38
  settings for, 36
  temperature, 36
  tension-free, 24
  ventilation, 36
  wall space, 37
  wholesome, 5, 35–47
Exercises, *see also* Movement
  and breathing, 44, 73, 92–96
  and fatigue, 50–51
  of individual body parts, 100–104
  integrative, 55
  and movement, 8
  for relaxation, 100–118
  sitting-up, 55–56
  skills in, 8
Equipment and furnishings, 38–47
  flexible arrangement of, 39–40
Excitability, 51
Eyes (turning inward), 4
Eyes-closed Story, 75–77

F

Fairy tales, 7
Family
  books about problems, 63–64
  disintegration of, 2
  instability of, 2
  problems of, 59–62

Fantasy, 4, 6, 7, 11
THE FAT BALLOON, 108–09
Fatigue
    and emotions, 51
    motor control and movement,
        50–51
    prevention of, 52
    resting to reduce, 72
    and skin, 50
    signs of, 50–52
    voice signals, 50
Fears, 61, 63, 65
Feedback (instant), 101
Feelings, see also Emotions
    acceptance of, 123
    "butterflies" in the stomach, 122
    constructive use of, 122
    developing control of, 6, 123–24
    expression of, 6, 17, 124
    games about, 124–132
    handling of, 120–133
    holding back of, 122, 133
    negative, 122
    outlet for, 122–124
    and palpitations of heart, 122
    and physical reactions, 17
    rapid breathing, 122
    recognition of, 122–123
    suppression of, 133
    and trust, 132
    universality of, 123
    vocabulary about, 123, 127, 130,
        131
Feingold, Ben, 13
Feingold Society, 13
Finger games, 78–80
Fine motor movements, see
    Movement
Flexibility in room arrangements,
    39, 40
FLIP-FLOP GAME, 14–16
THE FLOWER IN THE MEADOW IN
    THE MOUNTAIN, 96–97
Fluorescent lights, 36
THE FROGGIE, 107
Frustration, 13

G
Games (see also individual titles)
    arm movement, 78
    for communication skills, 24–33
    about feelings, 124–132
    finger, 78–80
    for relaxation, 99–118
GOLDEN FEATHER, 112–115
    extension of, 116–117
Gesturing, 9, 22
GENTLY FLOWS THE PLAYTIME
    NOW, 82
Golden Rule of Awareness, 6
Group
    awareness, 6
    harmony of, 116
    tension, 5
Groups
    active, 50
    anticipation for quiet, 53
    harmony of, 26
    in circles, 52
    mood of, 8
    normal, 50
    positions of children, 52–54
    standing or sitting, 54
GRASSHOPPER, GRASSHOPPER, 109

H
HAND SQUEEZE, 24
HANG LOOSE, 117–118
Harmony of group, 5, 26, 116
Health
    emotional, 17
    physical, 17
Heart beats, 92
Heart Breathe, see also Breathing
    exercises, 92–97
    as listening experience, 92
    as meditative experience, 92
    OH, LISTENING TO MY LOVE, 94
HEART BREATHE #1, 93
HEART BREATHE #2, 93–94
HEART BREATHE #3, 95
Heart (palpitations of), 122

Hemispheric integration of the
  brain, 11
Holding (calming effect of), 58
How Do You Do My Partner,
  26
Hugging (as emergency procedure),
  58
Hyperactivity, see Behavior,
  hyperactive
Humidity, 36–37
Humor
  gentleness of, 56
  and records, 33
  as relaxant, 56–58
  and silliness, 57

I

I Sit on the Floor, 117
I Woke Up One Morning, 68–69
If You're Angry, 126
Illness
  mental, 2, 3
  physical, 2
Imagery, 11
Imagination, 37
Imagination space, 37
Immaturity, 100
Infanticide, 3
Inner awareness, 4, 14, 73, see also
  Self-awareness
development of, 91–97
Inner self, 4, 73, 92
Insulin, 12
Integration (of brain hemispheres),
  11
Interpersonal relationships, 2, 7,
  16–17, 20–22, 24
Isolation, 40
  and emotional release, 58–59
Isometrics and Yoga, 100
It Was Time To Go To Bed, 83

J

Jiggling My Body, 110–111

K

Kinesthetic awareness, 101

L

Language skills, 5
Laterality
  cross-, 9–10
  and dominance, 8
Laughing (uninhibited), 51
Learning disabilities, 10
Lethargy, 11, 13
Letter to parents, 61–62
Life Crises events
  books about, 63–64
  comfort for, 59–62
Lighting (and environment), 36
Listening
  as demonstration of trust, 23
  to children, 20, 21
  as a two-way process, 22
  nonjudgmental, 22
  problems related to, 22–23
Loose arrangements, 53
Loose, see Hanging Loose
Low-stress program, 6
Lullabies, 82–83

M

Meditative experiences, see Heart
  Breathe
Mind (control of own), 11, 14
Minorities, 3
Mistrust, 2
Mood, 8
Motor activities, see Exercises;
  Movement
Motor abilities, see also Laterality
  screening for, 13
Movement, see also Exercises
  bilateral, 9
  categories of, 8–9
  control of, 5
  creative, 7

Movement *cont'd*
  cross-lateral, 9–10
  and fatigue, 51
  fine motor, 9
  learning through, 5
  nonlocomotor, 9
  and nonmovement, 8
  and pantomime, 33
  unilateral, 9
  whole body, 9
Muscular exercise
  overexertion, 54
  as relaxant, 65
  after sedentary periods, 55–56
Muscles
  control and release of, 100
  isometrics, 100
  overexertion of, 54
  relaxation of, 99–117
  release of tension in, 98–107
  small (use of), 9
  and Yoga, 100
Music
  lullabies, 82–83
  recorded, 80–81
  as relaxant, 80
  and songs, 80
  while painting, 85
Musical accompaniment, 8
Mutuality
  definition of, 6
  feelings of, 31
  and touching, 24

N

Names, use of, 78–79
Napping
  and dual-purpose room, 40–41
  environment for, 85–86
  need for, 10–11
  routine (importance of), 85, 87, 89
National Center for Health Statistics, 3

National Health Federation, 13
NATURE SEARCH GAME, 84
Nervous energy (use of clay to relieve), 45
News media, 2
Noise
  as cause of stress, 36
  as fatiguing, 51
Nonlocomotor movements, *see* Movement
Nonmovement, *see* Movement
Nonjudgmental approach, 22
Nonverbal communication, *see* Communication, nonverbal
Nonverbal conversations, 31–32

O

OH, LISTENING TO MY LOVE, 94–95
Open-ended programs, 10
Open space, 38
OUR OWN SPACE, 46–47
Overdiscipline, 3
Overtired, 49
Overindulgence, 3
Outdoor resting experiences, 71
  cloud watching, 84
  nature search, 84
  walking (after lunch), 86
  watching trees, 84–85
Oxygen, 73, 92

P

Pancreas, 12–13
Pantomime, 33
  to records, 33
Parents Anonymous, 63
Perceptual development, 13, 22
Perceptions (distorted), 2
Personality, 10
Physical
  disabilities, 3

Physical cont'd
  health, 16
Physical tiredness (signs of), 51
Pilgrims, 32
Pillows, 41
Place (alone), 41–47
Plasticine (therapeutic effect of), 45
Play-learning program, 6
Play
  alternating rhythms of, 72
  vigorous, 54
  vitality of, 1
Poisoning (lead or cadmium), 13
Pollution, 13
Postural positions, 100
Preservatives, 13
President's Commission on Mental
  Health, 3
Problems
  developmental, 14
  psychological, 8
  screening for, 8
  listening, 33
Program
  play-learning, 6
  low-stress, 6
  open-ended, 10
Protein, 12–13

Q

Quarrels
  handling of, 19
  the right to, 23
Questions to stimulate discussion,
  24, 31–32, 129
Quiet places, 41–47
  for resting, 118

R

Racial differences, 3
Rainbow Corner, 45–46
RAG DOLL, 118
Reconciliation process, 7

Recorded music, 80–81
Relationships (caring), 7
Relaxation, *see also* Rest, Napping
  atmosphere for, 1, 4
  and brain integration, 11
  body training for, 100–106
  cues for, 74
  environment conducive to, 16,
    40
  exercises for, 99–118
  and fatigue, 52
  and food, 59
  greatest single factor in, 17
  and humor, 56–58
  and music, 80–83
  and nonmovement, 8
  opportunities for, 12
  as opposite of tension, 100, 107
  and physical exercise, 100–106
  repetition for, 74, 78
  techniques for, 5, 52
Religious differences, 3
Remarriage, 2
Remediation
  programs, 8
  techniques, 14
Renewed energy, 7
Repetition (as relaxant), 74, 78
Respect, 6, 7
Rest, *see also* Relaxation, Napping,
    Sleep, Cots
  environment conducive to, 35–46
  exercises for, 54–56, 73
  and mental fatigue, 72
  outdoor times of, 71, 74, *see also*
    Outdoor resting experiences
  routine established for, 87
  short periods of, 72–74
  in sitting position, 73
  techniques for, 70–89
  wake-up time, 89
  warning of time for, 73
Resting mats, 74
RESTING TIME, 82
Rhythm of body, 10

Routine (importance of), 87
THE ROCK AND THE STREAM, 97
ROCKING, ROCKING, 95–96
Room arrangements, *see also*
    Environment
    bulletin boards, 37
    cardboard boxes for, 37, 41
    central, 39
    color in, 36
    dual-purpose room, 40
    flexible, 39–40
    imagination space, 37
    wall space, 7

S

Schedules (desirability for
    regularity of), 10
Screening for developmental
    problems, 8, *see also* Testing
Self, *see* Inner awareness, Inner self
Self-awareness, 6, 7, 9, 11, 92
Self-confidence, 3
Self-image, 14
Sensorimotor development, 13
Sensory output, 11
Serenity, 8
    abused child's need for, 63
    atmosphere of, 5, 62, 122
    definition of, 5
    environmental settings for, 36–37
    and human interactions, 20
    inner, 7
    and interpersonal skills, 39
    philosophy of, 37
SHAKE MY HAND, 25
SHOW ME FEELINGS, 125
Sinking places, 42
SILENT HOUR, 32
Silliness games, 57–58
Sitting-up exercises, 55
Skin (appearance of, and fatigue),
    50
Sleep, *see also* Napping
    environment for, 40

Sleep, *see also* Napping *cont'd*
    natural position of, 15
    need for, 87
    unhappy experiences of, 87
Smith, Lendon, 12–13
Socialization (opportunities for), 16
Socrates, 7
Songs (*see also* individual titles)
    improvising, 81–82
    lullabies, 82–83
    personalization of, 82
Space
    alone, 41–47
    imagination, 87
    open, 38
    wall, 87
Spatial relationships
    and brain integration, 11
    exercise in, 46–47
    OUR OWN SPACE, 46–47
    problems with, 8
Speech problems, 33
Staff, *see also* Teachers
    being open and honest with, 17
    working together, 16–17
Step-siblings, 2
Stimulation (need for), 11
Stories (*see also* individual titles)
    eyes-closed, 75–77
    repetition of, 74
Storytelling, 74–77
Stress and tension
    anticipation of, 50
    anxiety, 50
    and arm movements, 78
    benefits of, 3
    causes of, 18, 59–62
    and communicating with parents
        61
    constant state of, 122
    coping with, 7
    and deeper understandings
        between persons, 92
    destructive nature of, 122
    and family problems, 59–62

Stress and tension *cont'd*
  and fears, 60
  feelings and emotions, 17, 40,
    122–124
  generalized, 3
  irritability, 50
  meaningful use of, 5
  and natural development, 10
  reduction of, 5, 6, 40, 112
  related behavior, 10
  responding to, 48–69
  sources of, 2, 59–62, 63–69
  subliminal, 2
  symptoms of, 5
  tolerance level for, 17
  understanding of, 5
  unrelieved, 3, 4
  and weather, 64–69
Stress reduction (curriculum of), 5
Stroking (therapeutic effect of), 58
Sugar (as stimulant), 12

T

TALL TREES, 66
Tambourine accompaniment, 8
Tantrum (handling of), 58–59
Teachers, *see also* Staff
  coursework for, 4
  example of, 17
  interaction between, 16–17
Tables, 43–44
Tactile sensations, 42
Temperature in environment, 36,
  38
Temperament, 10
TEN LITTLE CHILDREN, 80
Tension, *see* Stress
Tent places, 42–43
Testing, 8, 14
THINK OF SOMETHING QUIET, 1,
  4, 20
Time of day (consideration of), 8
TIME TO REST, 79
Toilet (frequent use of), 11

TO TOUCH A STAR, 26
  variations of, 27–29
Touching
  as communication, 23–29
  games, 24–33
  importance of, 23
  and instant feedback, 101
  and mutuality, 24
  and tension-free environment, 24
  and toddlers, 23–24
Tranquility, *see also* Serenity
  and breathing exercises, 92
  and environment, 36
  and exercise, 115
  human striving for, 73
  joy of, 5
  mood for (establishing of), 72
  and resting, 73
Transition periods, 78
Tree watching activities, 84–85
Trust, 6, 7, 21, 23, 33, 132
TRUST WALK, 132–133
Turning inward, 4

U

Ulcers in children, 3
Unilateral movements, 9

V

Verbalization, 30
Visual discrimination, 8
Vocabulary
  feelings, 123
  Relaxation/tension, 107
Voice signals and fatigue, 50

W

WAKING, WAKING, LITTLE STAR,
  29
Weather
  consideration of, 8, 64
  extremes of, 64

Weather *cont'd*
  foggy, 67
  games about, 65–69
  rainy, 67–69
  as source of stress, 64–69
  stormy, 67–69
  windy, 65–66
WEATHER GAME, 64
Westman, Jack, 3
WHEN I'M ANGRY, 126

Whole body movements, 104–106
Wigwams, 43
THE WIND IS BLOWING ALL
    AROUND, 66
WINDY DAYS GAMES, 65–66

Y

Yoga, 100